THE
AMERICAN
MEDICAL
MACHINE

THE AMERICAN MEDICAL MACHINE

❖❖❖❖❖

Senator Abraham Ribicoff

with Paul Danaceau

Saturday Review Press

NEW YORK

Published simultaneously in Canada by
Doubleday Canada Ltd., Toronto.

Library of Congress Catalog Card Number: 74-154257

ISBN 0-8415-0200-5

Saturday Review Press
230 Park Avenue
New York, New York 10017

PRINTED IN THE UNITED STATES OF AMERICA

Design by Tere LoPrete

For Ruth, who experienced it all.

Acknowledgments

THERE ARE many doctors, hospital administrators, insurance officials, economists, and social scientists whose cooperation made this book a much easier task than it might otherwise have been. They spoke openly and honestly about the problems of American medicine without fear that admitting to weaknesses was in itself a sign of weakness. To them, I am grateful. But more particularly, I owe a deep debt to those who participated in the planning, the research, and the writing of this book.

Paul Danaceau brought a depth of knowledge and understanding, together with a familiarity with the subject, that gave this work much of its basic shape. Peter Ribicoff brought to the effort a sensitivity and a first-hand awareness of medical care that was invaluable. Finally, Rosemarie Wagner performed what is perhaps the most necessary but often most thankless part of any book, the hours of typing and preparing the manuscript. In addition, she could always be counted on to research a particular subject and ferret out important pieces of information when they were needed the most. She earned the respect of all of us, both for her ability and for her patience.

Contents

" . . . If we believe men have any personal rights at all as human beings, they have an absolute right to such a measure of good health as society, and society alone, is able to give them."

—ARISTOTLE

THE
AMERICAN
MEDICAL
MACHINE

Introduction

MY OWN PERSONAL experiences with doctors and hospitals have been few and far between. Outside of minor and routine illness and hospitalization, I have had little involvement with either. Whenever I did, it was always on the plus side. There wasn't a doctor who treated me that I didn't like personally or whose judgment and ability I did not fully respect and trust.

Other members of my family have had the same good fortune with regard to the quality of care they have received. They have not been so fortunate about the extent, the length, and the frequency of their illnesses, though.

Through their eyes and their experiences, I have seen, felt, and learned how excruciating sickness and disease can be; what it means to suffer, to be in pain and need medical help; and how vulnerable a patient or his family can be even under the best of medical conditions. I have seen how the red tape, the uncertainties, and the questions are difficult enough for a knowledgeable man. For the average man, perhaps not so knowledgeable about medical care, the barriers and doubts are heartbreaking, because nothing leaves a person or his family feeling so helpless as being sick and in need of medical care. That feeling exists when everything goes right, when the medical care is good and the atmosphere in which the care is provided is warm and compassionate. When this is not the case, then life for the sick and their families can be both terrifying and humiliating.

The late Eve Edstrom, a dear friend of mine who was the able and widely respected health and welfare writer for *The Washington Post*, sensed this. She died of cancer. On one of her last trips home from the hospital, she told her nurses and her friends that she wanted to write an article on what patients had to go through with the fragmentation of medical services. People who are sick, as she was at the time, she said, don't have the strength to arrange for their needs, to find a visiting nurse, a home-maker, or a practical nurse.

Yet so often in the American medical care system, the burden invariably falls on the sick. At the time in their lives when they are least able to fend for themselves, they are asked to do the most. Is it any wonder that people are frightened by our medical care system, fearful of hospitals, and fearful of doctors? Is it any wonder they won't challenge the system or ask the questions they should? Is it any wonder they will almost go down to their grave in ignorance rather than ask a question or demand the accountability they have a right to demand?

These are terrible wrongs that must be corrected. They are situations my family might have been trapped in had I been a factory worker or shoe salesman and not a United States senator who formerly was a governor and Cabinet secretary.

The illness and diseases that have afflicted my family were unusual. My wife, Ruth, suffered from a chronic circulatory system problem that affected her heart. She spent a good portion of the last years of her life in hospitals.

At first, she experienced severe and frequent nosebleeds, sometimes on a daily basis and losing as much as a cup of blood at a time. These were caused by abnormal swellings of blood vessels that were too close to the surface of her skin. In 1961, when I was Secretary of Health, Education, and Welfare in the Kennedy Administration, we learned of a surgeon at the Ohio State University College of Medicine, Dr. William H. Saunders, who had developed an operation to correct this problem. We went to Columbus, the operation succeeded, and for the first time since my wife was a little girl, she had relief from this discomfort and pain.

Some years later, we learned that there were swellings and shunts in blood vessels elsewhere in her body, particularly in her abdomen. The effect of this was a short circuit in her circulatory system that created an abnormal path for the blood flow and that eventually placed great stress on her heart. She tired easily. Hospitalization became frequent. So were blood transfusions. Round-the-clock private-duty nurses were a necessity. And during the last year of her life, alone, she was admitted to the hospital five different times.

Another member of my family, my son, Peter, who has a wife and two small children of his own and who lost a seven-week-old daughter in a sudden infant death in 1967, has had severe back problems most of his life. After years of his going to doctors, in which the problem was diagnosed variously as a slipped disc, a muscle spasm, and a bladder problem (these were all parts of the problem), an internist my son had been seeing, Dr. Morton Davidson, thought the symptoms warranted a visit to a neurologist.

It developed that Peter had a malformation of the veins and arteries imbedded in his spinal column, and that these were pressing against his nerves. Further diagnosis was needed, and the test—a spinal cord angiogram, in which dyes are injected into the veins to plot the exact location of the veins and arteries of the malformation— was almost as dangerous as the surgery he eventually underwent. But getting the angiogram wasn't as simple as it seemed. A National Institutes of Health team that had been performing them had just disbanded. A medical team was available at New York University Hospital, where Dr. Herbert Rubinowitz, a neurologist, was caring for Peter. But the necessary equipment had not been assembled. Time was important. Dr. Rubinowitz and Dr. Irvin I. Kricheff, a neuroradiologist, recommended that Peter fly to Paris so that Dr. René Djindjian, who had done more spinal cord angiograms than anyone else in the world, and with phenomenal success, could perform the angiogram.

After the angiogram, Peter flew immediately back to New York, where he was rushed from the airport straight to the hospital. Two days later, he was in surgery. It was a desperate operation, and we all knew it. We had the greatest admiration and respect for the neurosurgeon, Dr. Joseph Ransahoff, but he told us there were no guarantees. Peter might be paralyzed from the waist down. Without the surgery, however, there was no chance he would escape paralysis.

My son came out of the surgery without any paralysis of any kind. He did require a full year of rehabilitation and recovery, including six weeks in the outstanding Rusk Institute in New York (Institute of Rehabilitative Medicine of the New York University Hospital) learning to use his legs again. Now, about two years after the operation, he is again in good health.

I have no doubt that my wife and my son received the best medical care that was available, and that special care was rendered in our behalf, though I never asked for special treatment. And because I have good health insurance and am in the financial position to withstand the costs not covered by the insurance, I have been relatively unaffected by the cost of these two illnesses. But if I had the kind of health insurance most people have, and if I were in the financial circumstances most Americans find themselves in, I would have been unable to carry the burden. Certainly, I never would have thought of sending my son to Paris for a special diagnosis. As for Peter, he is a teacher; he earns a modest salary. He was lucky that during his year of rehabilitation he had a father upon whom he and his family could fall back.

As I said, the illnesses that my wife and son suffered, though not rare, still were fairly unusual. As such, had their care been less than adequate or their hospital experience less than satisfactory, their complaints might have been written off. I say this because frequently, when talking with doctors and hospitals, I have been told that a case in point was unusual or that the judgment of the patient and his family could not be trusted because they were too emotionally involved.

That argument is unacceptable. Of course the patient and his family are emotionally involved. Could anyone seriously expect it to be otherwise? Besides, the entire purpose of medicine, the whole ethic of medicine, is that the only important number is the number one: one patient, one doctor. That is the basis of the entire relationship. When that one patient doesn't count, when he can be written off, when his views can be discounted for whatever reason, when a problem exists that does not result in some serious introspection on the part of a hospital or a doctor because it is "only one case," then medicine is in serious trouble as a profession. And so are those of us who are patients.

This book is patient-oriented. It seeks to explain to the medical profession why patients are angry and frustrated and to explain to patients that there are very real and legitimate problems that doctors and hospitals face as well. All too often we take the easy way out of a tough problem by dealing in stereotypes; in this case, in simplistic notions of the abused patient and the indifferent doctor, just as twenty-five years ago, when medicine was at the peak of its prestige and status, we assumed that doctors could do no wrong and patients who complained were ingrates.

Though there is a strong critical tone to this book, this should not be interpreted as damning all of medicine or implying there is no possibility for improvement and reform. In its best sense, criticism is a form of analysis, not name-calling. It allows us to be specific about our complaints and the problems we seek to correct. And frequently criticism is most useful at precisely the moment when there is the hope and the prospect of change.

This is the point that I hope our nation has reached. There are many physicians who, along with the young people coming out of medical school today, form a nucleus within the medical profession that wants change as much as any critic on the outside. As a matter of fact, there isn't a criticism or a recommendation in this book that I have not heard from a doctor. Sometimes the comment was made privately, but it was made just the same. The critical stance holds, too, for the younger hospital administrators. As one doctor in his mid-forties said to me, "We were the silent majority of medicine for too many years. Now we realize we need to speak up and make our weight felt, or else the system won't change."

This is only the statement of one man, but I believe it represents a general attempt on the part of many within medicine to use the power they have to change American medical care.

But if doctors and hospitals need to change, that goes double for politicians and government officials. The whole history of government and medicine is one in which political leaders have consistently refused to speak up in the public interest. Only in the past several years has there been any real, strong appreciation of the fact that the American patients are a disenfranchised majority. Until then, the social history of American medicine could be reduced to a single phrase: don't disturb the doctors; or the hospitals; or the insurance companies. The time is long past for this country to show the same kind of concern for the rights of patients.

I do not have a quick and easy solution for every problem mentioned in this book. My respect for the problems is too great for such legislative glibness. Instead, it seems to me our most basic need is for a change of attitude, a new way of thinking about medical care, a philosophy that states our belief that to receive medical care is the individual's right, but to provide it is the nation's privilege.

I

Future Shock

As I stand before you on this day of April 20, 1980, I recall the year 1970, and wonder at all the changes that have occurred in the past decade. . . . The public used to be aghast when prognostications of costs of $100 per day were made, back in the late '60s and early '70s. What would they say to today's average of $400 per day, even in rural areas, with urban areas as high as $950 per day, and still going up?
From a speech by the late Mark Berke, executive director, Mount Zion Hospital and Medical Center, San Francisco, April 20, 1970.

FOR THE FAMILY of Norman W. Quynn, sixty-four, a retired grocer from Waynesboro, Pennsylvania, the future came early—ten years and two months early. They had their $1,000-a-day hospital bill on February 16, 1970, when they received a $4,599.90 bill for the four and a half days Mr. Quynn was a patient at the University of Pennsylvania Hospital in Philadelphia. He was admitted at 6 P.M. on a Sunday and died at 6:30 A.M. the following Friday.

Mr. Quynn underwent complex and extensive surgery for a bleeding ulcer that had hemorrhaged and for other stomach problems. His bill included the following items: room, $462; laboratory, $743; pharmacy, $114; operating room, $395; transfusions, $1,430; surgical-medical supplies, $321; radiology, $145; cardiology, $40; oxygen, $96; intensive care, $180; intravenous solutions, $139; breathing pressure machine, $20; pulmonary functions study, $60; albumin (a tissue-building substance), $320; other charges, $134.

The family was stunned by the size of the bill, especially since Mr. Quynn had previously spent the same amount of time in the local hospital at Chambersburg, Pennsylvania, where he had a kidney removed and received intensive care. The bill for those four and a half days was only $893, about $200 a day.

Other decades have become famous for scientific breakthroughs and advances in medical technology. The 1960s and 1970s will be remembered as the years when the sky was the limit in medical costs and nobody seemed to make much headway controlling them. In the 1960s alone, hospital costs almost tripled and doctors' fees nearly doubled. The average day in the hospital that cost $32.23 in 1960 cost $81.01 in 1970. The complete physical that cost $57 as recently as 1968 cost $100 in 1970. And six of every ten private dollars spent on medical bills came not from insurance programs but from the pockets of consumers.

More proof could be found in cities like Tulsa, Oklahoma, where medical bills accounted for 60 percent of all bankruptcies. Most involved young couples who had just bought a home, a car, and furniture. "You read through a lot of these cases," says attorney Ross Hutchins, "and you see things like a man owes Bank Americard $460. Then he owes the oil company $84. He owes the clothing store $185. The service station $30. The jewelers $25. And you say, 'Hell, that guy's problem wasn't medical.' Then you come to this. Pediatrics $104. Then you see he owes the hospital $195. Pathology laboratory $500. They'll let all the rest of those bills go bad because they've got a sick baby down there, and they've got to keep paying the money to keep that baby from being cut off without medical service and dying."

Or in Nashville, Tennessee, where Tom Moore, a consultant for prepaid group practice plans, has watched people lined up at a collection agency waiting to pay their medical bills. "They stand there, literally with their hats in their hands, paying off a few bucks at a time, promising to scrape up a few more next week," he says. "They're ashamed and fearful, afraid of missing a payment and afraid of change. It's an attitude of almost total servitude."

Thus, for millions of Americans, the symbol of medical care in the 1970s is not the Red Cross, the Blue Cross, or the physician's insignia. It is the dollar sign. It is also the doctor shortage, crowded facilities, and the devastating medical needs of the poor.

Even when they can afford a doctor, many people cannot find one. Nobody has kept count of how many thousands of towns, small communities, and neighborhoods have no doctor, but there are 134 counties in 36 states without one (according to the American Medical Association, which defines this as lacking "an active non-Federal physician"), and hundreds more with only one or two. When a town doesn't have a doctor, it tries every trick in the book. It puts up billboards, writes to medical schools, medical societies, and specialty organizations, advertises in medical journals, and builds a small suite of offices, which it offers rent-free, along with a house and a guaranteed income, to anyone who will come. When this doesn't work, they write to doctors in foreign countries, such as India or Colombia. And when even that fails, you are left with a town like Tilden, Illinois (population 1,000).

Tilden is one of 150 towns in Illinois without a doctor. Neighboring towns have them. One is so busy he won't see any new patients. The other can see only those who sign his daily registry before 8:30 A.M. The three doctors at a hospital five miles away are also overworked, as Tilden learned last year when an automobile struck a boy on a bicycle. He was rushed to the hospital, but all three doctors were out on call. The boy died the next morning. "I'm not a doctor and I can't prove anything," says Lawrence Campbell, the mayor of Tilden. "But I still feel that if that boy had immediate attention there might be some way of saving his life." Mr. Campbell himself took the boy to the hospital, waited fifteen minutes for a doctor to come, and then "got so mad I couldn't stand it so I just walked out."

That experience convinced the townspeople to buy a

new ambulance, one with a two-way radio so they could alert the hospital. But it's a doctor they really want, and the odds are against them. "Doctors just don't want to live here anymore unless they're from small towns and want to return," says Mayor Campbell. (In January of 1971, another Illinois town, London Mills, which has a population of 750, abandoned its twelve-year search for a doctor and said it would sell the $30,000 medical building it had put up in 1960.)

Royal Oak, Michigan, is an average middle-class suburb north of Detroit. Most of its 90,000 residents own their own homes and make a comfortable living. The community has 100,000 telephones, 26 churches, 22 schools, 4 movie theaters, 3 hotels, 2 banks, 2 golf courses, and a daily newspaper. It also has a 711-bed hospital, which services a large portion of Oakland County.

Like everything else in the county, William Beaumont Hospital is feeling the pressure of the area's rapid growth. In March of 1969, patients waited six or seven weeks for elective surgery. By January of 1971, they were waiting eight or nine weeks. So much emergency surgery has been showing up that two or three days a week the hospital postpones previously scheduled surgery for another week or two. Sometimes as many as ten cases a day are rescheduled.

Though not life-threatening, these situations cannot be shrugged off as minor inconveniences. People who have steeled themselves psychologically for surgery often find it difficult to go through the whole process again. "Cataracts are elective surgery and can be postponed," says Dr. Ivan Mader, the Beaumont chief of staff. "But a patient who can't see wants to be able to see without having to wait first nine weeks and then two more. A patient who has suffered bad burns and who needs skin grafts on a regular basis, and who is sixteen years old, as one of our patients is, does not suffer any physical harm when his grafts are postponed. But it sure interferes with his normal life, and he shouldn't have to go through it."

Whatever affluent suburbs like Royal Oak lack in hospital beds, they are supposed to make up in doctors. That's what popular wisdom says. But it doesn't apply for that scarcest of all medical creatures, the internist and family physician. Established internists already work a six-day, sixty-hour week, are booked up as far as three months in advance, are not seeing any new patients, and often are forced to send regular patients with immediate needs to the hospital emergency room. (Some people devise their own methods for beating the shortage and the waits. An Orlando, Florida, contractor, who had waited for more than an hour in his doctor's office, began to take his own temperature. A nurse rushed out and whisked him into an examining room.)

"I don't see any real hope of filling the gap between patient needs and the ability of the profession to supply those needs under current modes of operation," says Dr. Mader, who is himself an internist. "I would guess that 40 to 50 percent of what I do could be handled by a lay person, and it's well known that even more of a pediatrician's time could be turned over to people who could take a medical history and perform screening-type examinations like blood pressures and cardiograms to determine normal from abnormal. Then the physician could take over."

Physicians' assistants would help reduce the doctor shortage by forcing physicians to redefine their roles and use their time more efficiently. If the idea catches on and receives major financial support, they could become a substantial medical resource—but not for at least another ten years.

But it is the poor who are the most frequent victims of the nation's medical shortcomings. Compared to them, most people in this country have a medical smorgasbord.

Clifford Breaux, fifty-eight years old, of New Orleans, a Negro, owner of a small restaurant, unable to work for a year, is an example.[1] He was one of 30 million Americans admitted to a hospital in 1970. He made it on his ninth try. His medical problems were congestive heart failure and extreme overweight. He suffered severe body pains, had difficulty breathing, and could not digest his food. But one hospital refused to admit him five times, saying its beds were full, and three others turned him down because he didn't have the $200 deposit required for uninsured people. Finally, his wife and brother borrowed the money and he was admitted. Thirteen days later, he was dead.

1. Unsigned affidavit of Clifford Breaux, in *Rosezella Cook et al.* v. *Ochsner Foundation Hospital et al.*, U.S. District Court, E.D. Louisiana, 1970.

Mrs. Catherine Booker, forty-seven years old, also of New Orleans, a welfare recipient, is another example.[2] Her story is much the same. She had congestive heart failure, high blood pressure, and an acute and chronic asthma condition. Her sons tried to have her hospitalized nine times over a five-month period before they succeeded. One hospital turned her down eight times, again saying it lacked the beds. Another wanted a $325 deposit, which nobody in the family had. Then one night, gasping and semiconscious, she arrived by ambulance at a hospital that had refused her twice the same afternoon. She was admitted. But by this time she couldn't speak and had great difficulty breathing. An hour later she was dead.

There are many millions of Americans who go without any medical care or receive inadequate care because they are poor. They live in neighborhoods like the Del Paso Heights section of Sacramento, California, where there is no doctor for 30,000 people, or in the Kenwood-Oakland area of Chicago, where there are five doctors for 50,000.

In the absence of doctors, they turn to the most besieged medical facilities in the country: the overcrowded, understaffed, and underfinanced municipal hospitals. These hospitals often provide good care. But the potential for poor care is far greater here than elsewhere. Emergency-room waits of five to six hours are normal, and fourteen-hour waits are not entirely uncommon.

2. Affidavit of Edward Booker, in *Rosezella Cook et al.* v. *Ochsner Foundation Hospital et al.*

Even when the care comes, it often lacks any personal touch or sense of continuity. An infant girl was taken to Jacobi Municipal Hospital in New York City forty-four times during the first nine months of her life without ever being treated by the same physician twice. Another emergency room felt so pressured it refused to treat non-emergency patients.

Being admitted to a hospital is no guarantee things will get better for them. Medical records are frequently lost and overcrowding is so severe that cardiac patients are placed in halls near the nurses' stations. "You come to this hospital and we're telling you somebody's going to take care of you," says Dr. Seymour M. Glick, chief of medicine at New York's Coney Island Hospital. "The fact is, you may lie in a pool of feces, develop an ulcer, septicemia [blood poisoning], and perhaps ultimately die because of inadequate nursing care."

What the doctor shortage is to those outside the municipal hospital, the nursing shortage is to those inside it. "If you have one registered nurse and she is the only one covering three hundred patients, which is quite common in municipal hospitals, then some patients are going to die," says Dr. Glick. "In an intensive care unit, there should be one nurse for each two patients. I know of one which has one nurse for eleven patients. One was a young person in his twenties whose tracheostomy tube, through which he was breathing, became clogged up with his own secretions. With reasonable nursing care, he should have been suctioned every hour. But by the time the one nurse could get to him, he was dead. He

choked to death. They learned that at the postmortem.
I know another instance where a patient's tracheostomy
tube disconnected from his respirator and he died because there weren't enough nurses."

Even without preventable deaths, the nursing shortage results in some frightful situations in city-owned hospitals. A Los Angeles nurse says that when she is the only
nurse for seventy patients she can check on her patients
only once an hour if she has nothing else to do, which
means that medications are usually given late, and sometimes not at all. When she is tied up with one patient who
needs special care, she must rely upon aides who are not
highly trained to tell her if other patients are in trouble.
In her hospital, one third of all the medical ward patients
are weighed daily, and the rest every other day. Because
there is only one man to lift patients onto the scale, he
begins at 2:30 A.M. so he can finish by breakfast. The
maintenance men finish mopping the halls, loudly, at
12:30 A.M. At about 5 A.M., nursing aides begin taking
temperatures in order to finish in time to pass out medications before breakfast. So patients are wakened at
12:30 A.M., around 2:30 A.M., 5 A.M., and 6 A.M. on a
normal night.

Then there are the rural poor, like the migrant workers. For them, medical care means driving fifty or a hundred miles to a hospital; crossing back into Mexico,
where medical care is cheaper and "more humane"
(these are United States citizens); watching infants run
up life-threatening fevers because nobody has the $10
charged by the local doctor; and having a hospital say

after childbirth: "You pay the bill or we keep the baby."
Almost every child, says Dr. Raymond M. Wheeler, a
Charlotte, North Carolina, internist who has followed
the trail of the migrants, grows up with some preventable
physical defect or disease. On one trip, Dr. Wheeler
stopped at the one-room shelter where six children lived
with their parents.

"On the bed lay a three-month-old infant," he said in
testimony before the Senate Subcommittee on Migratory
Labor. "It was emaciated, restless, wailing, and occasionally pulling at a bottle which we soon discovered contained sour milk. There was no refrigerator in which to
keep formula. The child had been ill for weeks, according to its mother, but at its last visit to the clinic, a day
or two earlier, no medication had been prescribed. A
very quick examination disclosed pus pouring from its
right ear. We made arrangements for the child to have
penicillin and individually packaged feedings of formula
which the mother could not afford. I suspect we were too
late, and I doubt if the child survived. . . .

"I remember vividly the shock I received when one
young boy was brought in who was well-nourished and
I touched his skin—warm, soft, resilient—unlike any I
had seen all day, and I called to the student with me to
come and put his hand on that child in order that he
might refresh his memory of what a healthy skin feels
like."

This is part of the reason why, although the United
States spends more money on medical care than any
other country—more than $80 billion a year and over

$350 per person (migrants receive $20 worth of medical care a year)—fourteen other nations do a better job of preventing infant deaths. Twenty years ago, only six nations had a better record. Forty of each 1,000 black male babies born die before their first birthday, nearly twice the national average. For Alaska Indians, the rate is 56, even though deaths among American Indian babies dropped 48 percent since 1955.

Poor housing and other environmental conditions contribute to infant disease and death. But poor housing has nothing to do with the fact that each year one million children are born to women who receive no medical care during pregnancy or delivery and sometimes both. That is strictly a medical problem. And when doctors are scarce, facilities overcrowded, and nobody in medicine or government assumes responsibility for coordinating the medical needs of children and their families on a community-wide basis, it is almost inevitable that infant deaths will rise.

Other countries, especially Finland and Sweden, offer free cribs or cash bonuses as incentives for prenatal care. In America, however, the poor often feel stigmatized by free care. "Doctors think you have to take their insults because they're giving you everything free," said one woman in describing the care she and her infant had received at an outpatient clinic. "I sit there, looking at the dirty walls, and wonder why I'm there."

All any patient really wants is some assurance that he will find a doctor when he needs one, that he will receive high-quality care at a cost he can afford, that his rights as a consumer will be respected, and that none of this will depend upon his job, his income, his neighborhood, or the color of his skin.

Whether he receives such assurances, though, is a matter of pure luck, because most of this country's medical care systems, such as they are, have been organized more for the convenience of the providers—doctors, hospitals, and insurance carriers—than for the needs of the consumers. No matter how frustrating this has been to those providers who want to improve medical care, it is insignificant compared to the hardships suffered by patients. For it is the patient who is the ultimate victim of the fact that medical care in America is a private business and not a public responsibility. It is the patient who goes without medical care. It is the patient who receives inadequate medical care. It is the patient who comes to believe that medical care is a luxury and that "most doctors don't want you to bother them," as nearly seven of every ten did in a national poll reported in 1968.

Just finding medical care can be both a mystery and an endurance test for even the most sophisticated consumer. He never knows what will happen at any point along the way and usually winds up going to at least five different places. He must find a pediatrician for his children, an obstetrician-gynecologist for his wife, an internist for general medical problems, a general surgeon whenever that is required, and perhaps a specialist or two. When an emergency arises, he forgets about all of them and heads straight for the hospital. If people had to go through that to get their automobiles serviced and repaired, they would take to the streets in protest. But they accept this as normal for medical care.

Staying clear of backbreaking medical bills also is more luck than anything else. Where a man lives, works, and how much he earns—rather than any personal feelings he might have on the matter—usually determine the kind of medical insurance he and his family have. If he belongs to one of many unions for whom medical benefits follow right behind wages as a bargaining point, he has less to fear. But if he has nobody to organize and articulate his medical needs, he can wind up paying $20 of his $400-a-month salary (before taxes) on insurance that is limited to $400 for surgery and $40 a day for a hospital bed.

Once he is in a plan, he learns about the small print. Twenty-one of seventy-five Blue Cross plans, according to the most recent government survey, still do not fully cover laboratory services. Radium therapy, so important to cancer patients, is covered in full by only six plans and not at all by fifty-seven. A dozen plans don't cover blood transfusions, and another twelve cover them only partially. Twelve more don't cover X rays, six cover them partly, and sixteen occasionally. Commercial policies often reject maximum limits that are more favorable to consumers and pay on a piecework basis instead. One policy allows $10 for X rays that can cost as much as $40; $15 for oxygen, which can run as high as $100; and $25 for blood transfusions that often cost $50.

Waiting periods between the time a person joins a plan and the time he is eligible for some benefits take another bite out of the security the consumer thinks he has bought. Colorado subscribers suffering from gall bladder problems and ulcers of the stomach have to wait eleven months or foot the full cost of the bill themselves. The New Hampshire–Vermont plan won't cover hernias, varicose veins, or any female genital problem for nine months. Full maternity benefits do not begin in fifty-eight plans until *after* nine months, and sometimes ten, have passed. Infants are not covered in ten plans until they are two weeks old.

Applied to the nation as a whole this means that one of every six people under sixty-five has no hospital insurance, the basic ingredient in any insurance package. That's 30 million Americans. One in five is without surgical insurance (35 million). One in four is not covered for extra in-hospital medical expenses, such as doctors' visits (46 million). Half the population has no X-ray and laboratory insurance outside the hospital (89 million). Roughly the same number of people are unprotected against the rising cost of prescription drugs (85 million). And 90 percent has no insurance against dental expenses (164 million).

In short, the consumer is left at the mercy of a profession (medicine) and an industry (hospitals and insurance) that answer only to themselves, and of a marketplace that cannot effectively guarantee that his medical care needs will be met, both in terms of actual services and financial protection against the skyrocketing cost of care.

Patients who must deal with this system, which means almost everyone, are not interested in learning what American medicine has accomplished for them in the past twenty-five years. They just want to make sure they don't become its victims in the next twenty-five years.

CHAPTER

II

Where Have All the Doctors Gone?

WHEN GARY RINKER, the eighteen-year-old son of a Clayton, New Mexico, rancher, fell and fractured his spine in October of 1969, he was rushed to the local hospital, a fully equipped, thirty-five-bed institution built in 1962 to meet all the medical needs of the 10,000 people who live in and around Clayton.

But between the time the hospital was built and the time of Gary Rinker's accident, the medical situation in Clayton had changed dramatically. The town, which had five or six doctors throughout the 1950s and the early 1960s, was down to only one. And he couldn't apply a body cast. So Gary Rinker was placed in splints and taken by ambulance to the nearest hospital outside of Clayton. It was in Amarillo, Texas, some 135 miles away.

That was just a start. Twice in the next eight months

Clayton ran out of doctors altogether, and Union County Hospital had to close its doors and transfer all its patients to Amarillo. People with routine medical needs began driving a hundred miles for an office visit. Those who needed surgery or hospitalization for serious medical problems either drove the 135 miles to Amarillo or flew 300 miles to Albuquerque.

The hospital reopened in the fall of 1970, when the townspeople attracted a former medical missionary to the area. And though the people of Union County no longer drove a hundred miles for an office visit, they nonetheless had to choose betwen Amarillo and Albuquerque for surgery or major hospitalization. Because a one-doctor hospital, as administrator Howard Conley pointed out, really couldn't do much more than provide first aid. Surgery was out, since both New Mexico state law and the regulations of the Lutheran Hospitals and Home Society of America, which runs the hospital, require two doctors in the operating room. And complex medical problems were also beyond the range of a one-man institution.

What happened in Clayton has been happening all over rural America. It's an old, familiar script. A town loses its doctors through death and retirement; younger men move in but leave in six months because they never have a day off and are unable to spend any time with their families; others stay away altogether because they can't take the professional isolation of being not just the only doctor in town but the only one for miles around; and, in Clayton's case, something extra, one doctor whose license was revoked by the state board of medical examiners because he was a narcotics addict.

The script is just as familiar in the urban areas. Walk into any hospital emergency room on any given day and the chances are that at least one third of the people waiting to be seen, and perhaps as many as two thirds, won't have the kind of serious problem that emergency rooms are supposed to handle. They will be there because it's the only place they can find a doctor.

If they are poor, they have come because they probably have no doctor at all. If they are middle-class, they may not have a doctor either, especially if they are new in town. Some will be there because their doctor is too busy to see them that day. And still others because it is a weekend, an evening, or a Wednesday afternoon and they don't know what else to do when they can't reach their regular physician.

Though they eventually receive care, it's the wrong way to get it. The emergency room is twice as expensive as a doctor's office, is twice as impersonal, and has few preventive measures. The person who is treated today could just as easily be back tomorrow or the following week. But when the demand for medical care exceeds the supply and the availability of doctors, what other choice is there?

There isn't much choice in a city like Rochester, New York, where for the past four years the Monroe County Medical Society has been averaging fifty phone calls a day from people looking for a doctor, but where 90 percent of the society's membership isn't taking any new patients. So people settle for part-time medical care. They find a pediatrician who can see the newborn baby but not the older children, or one who can see the sick child but can't give the healthy youngster a checkup. One woman who moved to a Rochester suburb became so frustrated in her efforts to find a doctor for her husband, who had a fever of 104 degrees, that she drove him forty miles to see their old doctor in the town they had just left.

What Rochester and most other communities are feeling is not just the pressure of an overall doctor shortage —the federal government estimates the country is roughly 50,000 physicians short—but the shortage of a particular kind of doctor, the internist, pediatrician, and family practitioner who offers what has come to be known as "primary" care. He is the key to it all, the heart of the modern medical care system. He is the man you automatically turn to when you are sick, who takes you in, hears your story, diagnoses your illness, treats you when he can, or guides you through the often bewildering maze of specialty medicine when you need something else. He is part physician, part confidant, and part psychiatrist.

At least, that is how it is supposed to work.

Except that the more specialized American medicine became, the less attractive medical students and physicians found primary care and family practice. People who chose this less dramatic career line were viewed, and often still are, as medicine's second-class citizens, unable to make the grade in the more "challenging" fields, not bold enough for surgery or brilliant enough for research.

"We weren't told anything directly," recalls a doctor who finished medical school in the early 1960s, "but the message came through loud and clear just the same. You could spend your time treating the routine medical needs of people if you wanted to. That was your business. But the real excitement, the prestige, the honors, and the rewards weren't in being an L.M.D. [local medical doctor]. They were in specialization and research. That's where all the action was. Sometimes you almost thought that the most prestigious claim any M.D. could make was that he had never treated the same patient twice in his entire professional life."

Both tendencies—to go into academic research and to specialize—have done more than affect the ability of patients to find primary care. They have also created barriers for specialists who have had to recruit additional help, such as Dr. Robert B. Jeffrey, a Phillipsburg, New Jersey, radiologist.

From July of 1969 until January of 1971, a period of eighteen months, Dr. Jeffrey searched for a replacement for one of his two partners at Warren Hospital, a 250-bed general hospital serving the 75,000 residents of Warren County. His experience was fairly typical of the problems anyone in search of a doctor is likely to encounter.

His first move was to write off any graduate of a foreign medical school who was not a United States citizen because his malpractice carrier would not cover them, and because it takes five to six years to become a naturalized citizen. Others were excluded because, in the registry provided by the American College of Radiology, they had expressed a preference to practice in certain sections of the country or in certain individual states.

He sent a mimeographed job description notice to 200 likely candidates. Ten answered. Some didn't want to live in a community of only 18,000. Others felt that the salary was insufficient. Dr. Jeffrey was offering $40,000 a year to start and $60,000 (his current salary) within three years. When Dr. Jeffrey began practicing in 1951, the starting salary was $9,000. He has since watched the basic starting salary for radiologists go to $12,000 in 1952, $20,000 in 1958, $30,000 in 1963, and $40,000 today.

"If you want someone with experience, then $40,000 is your minimum," says Dr. Jeffrey. "If a fellow can get a job at $45,000 or $50,000 in a slightly less desirable area, then he is not going to take $35,000 or $40,000 in a more pleasant place."

Although nobody said why $40,000 was not enough, Dr. Jeffrey felt that the cost of medical education might be one factor. Not infrequently, young doctors finishing their residencies are so heavily in debt that job choices are made on a flat financial basis. A survey of medical students made in 1964 showed that although they generally came from affluent backgrounds, one of every three had taken at least one loan to meet his expenses. One in ten had received loans from three separate sources, and one in eight said he didn't have enough money at mid-year to get through. By 1967, two of every five students had taken a loan, and their average debt was $3,046. Graduating seniors owed an average of $4,400.

Once, when Dr. Jeffrey thought he finally had found somebody, a background check showed that the man was an alcoholic.

His next step was to talk with radiology residents at medical schools in Philadelphia, which is an hour and a half from Phillipsburg. None was available. Most were staying in academic medicine or continuing their residencies, choosing, as Dr. Jeffrey put it, "the apparent security of the ivory tower." And he understood why they had made that choice.

In academic medicine, he says, the physician is free from the time-consuming business side of medicine. He doesn't have to get involved in intricate billing procedures, recruiting ancillary personnel, replacing equipment, expanding the physical plant, or many other problems that come up on a day-to-day basis.

They also have more time to themselves. "A crew of residents covers the teaching institution at night, on holidays, and part of the weekends," he says. "When there were three of us at Warren Hospital, our work week averaged seventy hours a week. This includes on-the-job coverage 365 days of the year. It is difficult to practice with two radiologists, and almost an impossibility for one to cover the department for any length of time. With three, we can manage to get in one or two scientific meetings a year and plan on two or three weeks of vacation a year."

When Dr. Jeffrey took five days off in the fall of 1970

to interview possible candidates in Chicago, it was the first time off he had taken in twenty months. More and more physicians are becoming sensitive to the hours they work, especially when they look around them and see that, among physicians, divorce and heart disease are increasing, while the rest of society is emphasizing leisure time and heading toward a thirty-five-hour work week. Physicians who leave their offices in the community for academic or hospital-based medicine frequently seek more "interesting" cases. But basically they want a situation in which they can practice medicine satisfactorily and still have relatively normal hours and a decent family life.

Finally, Dr. Jeffrey encountered the problem of the superspecialists. Whereas there were only thirty-four recognized specialties several years ago, there are now sixty-four. To the resident in pediatric radiology, neuroradiology, radiology therapy, or nuclear medicine, Robert Jeffrey is a general practitioner. The new breed is focusing on more-narrow areas, partly as a result of further developments and refinements in medical science and partly, it seems, out of a sense of self-protection. Some told Dr. Jeffrey that since various accountability factors such as peer review and recertification or relicensing were just around the corner, they would be in a more secure position if they set definite limitations on the scope of their practice.

This sense of self-protection is openly acknowledged by both the older and younger generations of physicians when they talk about the rise in malpractice suits and the price of malpractice insurance, and how it is affecting the supply of doctors and the actual practice of medicine.

Many physicians insist that the high cost of malpractice insurance will soon force them and their colleagues out of practice. Malpractice claims are increasing rapidly and $100,000 judgments and settlements are not unusual. But, for the moment, doctors are not leaving practice. Instead, they are thinking twice about the procedures they undertake (which may have a salutary effect), where they practice, and whom they see.

Dr. Martin Spector, a Philadelphia ear-nose-throat specialist, won't see patients that his nurse, who has been with him twenty-five years and who takes the medical history, regards as likely to sue. "It is impossible to get 100 percent results in medicine as well as in any other field," he says, "and we won't take the case of a patient who wants guarantees." Without the fear of a lawsuit, he probably would treat these patients.

Physicians in the high-risk specialties of anesthesiology, neurosurgery, and orthopedic surgery sometimes shy away from practicing in New Mexico, California, or Washington, D.C., where their premiums have skyrocketed. The cost of malpractice insurance was partially responsible for two physicians, a surgeon and an obstetrician, staying in Pennsylvania instead of moving to Clayton, New Mexico, the town that has been limping along with one general practitioner for the past few years. Malpractice insurance would have cost them together $6,000 a year in New Mexico compared to the $1,500 they were paying in rural Pennsylvania. A neurosurgeon who chooses to practice in Los Angeles must pay $2,900 for the same coverage that cost him $780 in 1969. An orthopedist who wants to establish himself in Washington, D.C., must pay $1,380 for coverage that would have cost $608 two or three years ago.

Apparently arbitrary decisions by insurance companies in canceling malpractice coverage have almost forced older physicians, who may never even have had a claim made against them, out of practice. This happened to one general practitioner in Cambridge, Massachusetts, who learned about this in time for the Massachusetts Medical Society to place him with another carrier.

He is the kind of physician the country can least afford to lose, because it's primary care that people need the most. But there aren't enough primary care physicians to go around. There are only 16,500 pediatricians available to treat the nation's 58 million children under 15 years of age, a ratio of 1 pediatrician for every 3,500 youngsters. Among internists, who are replacing the general practitioner as the closest thing to a "family" doctor that the country has, the ratio is far worse. It's 1 doctor for every 4,080 people, whereas most experts feel a 1 to 750 ratio is best for good continuous primary care. Furthermore, like every other kind of physician, these men and women are distributed unevenly throughout the population. One quarter of the nation's entire supply of internists and pediatricians can be found in two states—California and New York.

The closer one looks, the worse it gets. Though both the cities and the suburbs have been losing primary care physicians at a regular rate as specialization has increased, those that are available have congregated in the more affluent neighborhoods. No surprise, perhaps, until one looks at the numbers. In Chicago there are more private doctors in a single North Shore medical building than in the entire West Side poverty area of some 300,000 Negroes, and more doctors' offices in an affluent North Side community than in the South Side poverty ghetto where 400,000 people are living. In Boston, at one time, the most affluent 40 percent of the population laid claim to 90 percent of the city's internists, pediatricians, and obstetricians.

Those private doctors who are available to the poor generally are not the best. "Many of these physicians are in the slums because they cannot make the grade in a middle-class neighborhood, because of discrimination, inexperience, incompetence or senility," says Pierre DeVise, a DePaul University sociologist who has studied slum medicine in Chicago. "Some are too weak or old to move. And these physicians can do little more than give shots and prescribe pills."[1]

In such circumstances, patients frequently wind up on a medical assembly line. Half a dozen children with high fevers are treated in the same room. Patients are billed for answers to questions about family members who are at home (charges the same physician would never ask his more affluent patients to pay, if he has any). One clinic

1. Pierre DeVise, et al., *Slum Medicine: Chicago's Apartheid Health System* (Community and Family Study Center, University of Chicago, January 1, 1969), p. 20.

director, who describes himself as a "battlefield medic" and insists that "each patient is considered individually," sees an average of one hundred patients a day. That's less than five minutes per patient if he works an eight-hour day and a flat six minutes per patient if he works ten hours. Medical students who have observed him in action report that he doesn't even wash his hands between examinations.

Another ghetto physician in Chicago became so proficient at telephone medicine that he continued his practice while in the army. He was stationed in Arkansas. By using long-distance phone calls and weekend passes, he treated 475 patients one month and 715 the next.

These are the experiences of people who *do* see a doctor. Thousands more, perhaps millions, do not, and nobody really has a clear idea how extensive or serious that unmet medical need actually is. If Montgomery, Alabama, is an accurate barometer, then 88 to 92 percent of the poor (both black and white) are not receiving any medical care at all when they are sick or are receiving it much later than they should. On any given day in Montgomery, a city of 133,000, about 120 to 150 poor people will need medical care, but only 10 will receive any, according to a University of Alabama Medical School survey. The older people will have chronic illnesses like heart disease, high blood pressure, and diabetes, while the children will have infections, influenza, ear trouble, and skin disease, for the most part.

There are various reasons why they never see a doctor. Many are the poorest in the city and can't afford the cost of public transportation, let alone the cost of an office visit. Others are put off by earlier experiences at a local clinic. They never saw the same doctor twice, and when they did, he was always in a frantic hurry. "This was a man who was giving of his private hours, his private patients were waiting for him, and, you know, he turned up and saw as many as he could and vanished again," said Dr. Peter Peacock, chairman of the medical school's Department of Public Health and Epidemiology.

Nursing and clerical help frequently made patients feel unwanted because they couldn't pay, and the patients decided that no matter how sick they became, they wouldn't go back. "The lesser-level help in the office made them feel like dirt with remarks like 'You don't think we're going to put ourselves out for you, do you?' " Dr. Peacock said.

The doctor shortage of the 1970s is hardly a recent development. It has been building up for some forty years, ever since an editorial in the August 27, 1932, issue of the *Journal of the American Medical Association* (*JAMA*) suggested that perhaps the time had come for the medical profession to practice "professional birth control."

"The United States," said the editorial, "already has more physicians in proportion to its population than any other country in the world; if this ratio is still further increased, it is evident that an oversupply of doctors threatens, with an inevitable lowering of the standards of the profession. Perhaps there is need for professional birth control."

What the editorial did not say was that the income of physicians had dropped almost 40 percent between 1919 and 1932 and that it was going to drop even more the next year. Maintaining high standards of medical care may have been the announced intention of the AMA, but protecting the economic position of doctors clearly seems to have been the underlying motive. The Federation of State Medical Boards admitted as much a few years later when it spoke of the "other beneficial results [that] are becoming evident" in the new policy, such as 10,000 fewer doctors over the next twenty years, a development whose "implication . . . on the welfare of the future practitioner is evident."

But the issue of motivation was largely irrelevant, because the 1930s marked the beginning of medicine's heyday as a private business. It was a time when the concept of a public voice in determining the supply and availability of doctors didn't even exist. What the doctors wanted, the doctors got. And they were looking forward to a time "not far distant," as AMA President Dr. Walter L. Bierring said in 1934, when the medical needs of the population could "effectively" be met by only half the doctors then in practice. Clearly, medicine belonged to the physician and everybody else had to accept that fact whether they liked it or not.

The proof was in the success of "professional birth control." Within five years, medical schools had cut their enrollment some 18 percent. And the cuts stayed, because the schools did not reach their 1933 level of accepting 7,500 students a year again until 1951, almost twenty years later.

Yet in retrospect, the crucial years were not the 1930s, though they severely limited the capacity of the nation's medical schools. They were the post–World War II years of 1948 to 1950 when progressive medical educators began looking at the postwar birth rate and saw, for the first time, that the country was going to be perhaps 40,000 doctors short by 1960. They were not alone. A presidential adviser made the same prediction. So did the Public Health Service.

The reformers' appetite had been whetted by the fact that the country had just emerged from the experience of turning out an additional 7,000 doctors during the wartime years by reducing medical school to three years, admitting students every nine months, and taking in more students. If the country could do this for a war-time emergency, then why not for a peacetime emergency?

But the old ways prevailed. The AMA would have none of it. Consequently, neither would the Congress, which was still afraid to assert itself on any continuing basis in this field. If the war was over, the emergency was over. It was time to return to normal. And normal to the AMA meant limited federal aid to stabilize the financial position of existing medical schools but no federal aid, or as little as possible, to increase enrollments. One had to be wary of the "unknown implications and consequences of Federal aid." Besides, that old demon of "professional standards" was still lurking about. But if these were a principal concern, why establish a self-policing mechanism that operated, of all places, at the original source of supply? Far better results could be achieved by visits to medical schools by the AMA's own Council on Medical Education, which had the power of accreditation.

And so it went. In 1951, the AMA's Bureau of Medical Economics Research spoke of "a surplus or a potential surplus" of doctors. Four years later, in 1954, the bureau said the basic problem wasn't numbers; it was distribution, and the country only needed another 361 physicians to set that straight. Finally, in 1958, the AMA cautiously acknowledged the doctor shortage, but it took another nine years before the AMA called, in 1967, for the "immediate and unprecedented increase" in medical enrollment others had been urging as early as 1948.

The net result of these developments was that when the federal government estimated that the country was short 50,000 doctors as of February, 1971, the nation could look back and see that its medical schools had turned down some 100,000 qualified applicants alone between 1960 and 1970. Not enough places.

The whole situation might have been much worse had not the federal government finally begun to carve out a role for itself in medical education in 1963 and made construction grants available to medical schools. Whatever progress was made in turning out more doctors during the 1960s can be attributed directly to Washington.

But in terms of current need, federal efforts came too late and offered too little. Washington never really provided, on any continuing and substantial basis, the cash for day-to-day operations, teachers' salaries, and equipment that the medical schools desperately needed. Nor did it provide enough of what the medical student needed: scholarship and loan money.

One clear result of this failure has been the small numbers of blacks, Puerto Ricans, Mexican-Americans, American Indians, and orientals in medicine. Whether they would provide medical care to their own people after medical school is open to question, but until more than 5.8 percent of all medical students come from minority groups, it's a moot question.

A larger result is that the full effect of federal programs from fiscal years 1969 and 1970 will be to produce —by 1975 at the earliest—another 1,600 doctors, an increase of slightly more than one-half of one percent of the current physician population of 318,000. If they follow the patterns of their predecessors, then about one of every six won't even practice medicine, but will go into teaching, research, administration, and industry, and some will drop out of medicine altogether. And if those who actually practice medicine follow the same patterns of specialization and geographic distribution, only certain groups and sections of the country will benefit.

For example, one paradox of the current manpower situation has been that since so much of medicine's mystique and financial rewards are geared toward surgery, the country has produced a surplus of surgeons. Thus, while many internists work sixty and seventy hours a week and are booked up three months in advance, some surgeons still in their thirties are living in semi-retirement.

Dr. Lionel Zuckerbraun of Los Angeles is one of them. Early in 1971, about fourteen months after he returned from Vietnam, Dr. Zuckerbraun began looking around to see if there was a city of about 50,000 that needed him more than Los Angeles. He hasn't found one.

Sometimes he works only ten hours a week. "My wife sees me sitting around the house at two in the afternoon or playing catch with my son and wonders what's going on," he says. "But they don't really need me here. I'm thirty-seven years old, I'm at my peak, and all I'm really doing is filling in my days creating a demand for myself by becoming friends with John Doe, M.D., so that after months of lunches, hockey games, and golf, he thinks of Lionel Zuckerbraun when he sees someone who needs a thyroid operation. Sometimes it can be a very pleasant existence doing nothing, because you can make $36,000 a year by doing only five or six operations a month. But mostly, I feel I'm wasting my time. There must be hundreds of guys like me but they won't admit it."

Meanwhile, American's medical schools are on the financial rocks. In a sense, they always have been. Medical schools traditionally were not paying propositions. Outside money, both private and from the more profitable departments within the university, actually supported many of them. And when, in the spring of 1970, money was tight and the outside funds dried up, education costs went up and the universities didn't have the extra cash lying around, and the federal government cut back on the research grants to which schools had become accustomed, 43 of the country's 107 medical schools screamed for help and received "financial distress" grants from Washington.

They're not in much better shape now. Many can see only two or three years ahead. They are, as the Reverend Robert J. Henle, president of Georgetown University in Washington, D.C., told a House subcommittee, "gambling on a Federal program, a state program, or an act of God." At a state-supported medical school in the Midwest, the dean says, "You don't know what trouble really is until you try and get the legislature to put more money into a medical school that sends 75 percent of its graduates to other states." And at Saint Louis University they closed the dental school to keep the medical school open, a tradeoff that prompted Dr. Robert H. Felix, the medical school dean, to remark that "we're living off our own flesh."

This, then, is where the nation stands with regard to medical manpower: not enough doctors; those we have unevenly distributed by specialty and geography; federal programs that are insufficient to deal with the basic supply problem; medical schools foundering financially; the country on the verge of a national health insurance program that probably will unlock an even greater demand for physicians' services; and those who at the moment seem to be holding the whole system together, the emergency room physicians, saying they can't hold out much longer.

"We've reached our limit," warns Dr. Milton N. Luria, education director in the emergency department of Strong Memorial Hospital in Rochester, New York. Like nearly every other emergency room in the country, Strong Memorial treated twice as many patients in 1970 as it did in 1960. (Nationally, there were some 43 million visits to emergency rooms in 1970, as compared with 9.4 million visits in 1954.) And like every other physician who is providing this care, he finds little satisfaction in the increased patient load.

"Should we congratulate ourselves for being ahead when we are so far behind?" he asks. "The emergency room is a safety valve and all it really does is cover up the full extent of the manpower shortage elsewhere." What particularly troubles Dr. Luria is that patients who once tried to telephone a doctor before coming to the emergency room (he once treated a patient who made eighteen phone calls to find a doctor), don't even do this anymore. "They know it's tight, so they just come to us," he says.

If Dr. Luria had his way, everyone in Rochester would have a personal physician available to him at all times, as he and his six partners in internal medicine are to their patients. Somebody is always on call 24 hours a day, 365 days a year, so that, if the patient's personal physician is unavailable, another member of the group will respond. Patients are encouraged to call at night and on weekends, and the partners are not disturbed by the fact that patients could frequently get through the night without seeing anyone. "A major part of the physician's job is to give reassurance." says Dr. Luria. "The problem may be small to us but it's terribly important to the patient. Just the laying on of hands may give him a good night's sleep." And a colleague of his, Boston pediatrician Dr. Joel J. Alpert, castigates his fellow physicians who complain that 50 to 75 percent of the patients they see just need someone to talk to by asking, "What do you think medicine is all about?"

Actually, that's the whole issue: what *is* medicine all about? What constitutes good medical care? Who is receiving it and who is not? And whose responsibility is it to make the necessary changes, either by increasing the number of doctors and physicians' assistants or by creating new forms of organization and delivery?

Probably no community in the country has ever seriously asked itself these questions. Nor has the federal government. To the extent that they have been asked at all, they have been asked—and resolved—by the medical profession itself; not through any conscious process of assessing how the profession could best meet the medical needs of the population, but through the private choices of individual physicians in deciding the specialty they would enter, where they would practice, and how they would practice.

That may have been satisfactory for an earlier time, a simpler time. It still may be good enough in some places and for some specialties. But providing a basic human need for 208 million people in the medically and socially complex decade of the 1970s clearly ought to rest on something more substantial than the personal preferences of 318,000 independent entrepreneurs.

III

The Cost Victims:

How Many Are Enough?

EVERY YEAR SINCE about 1961, an average of 18,500 Americans have decided they would rather live in Canada than in the United States. While most have left this country because of poor job opportunities, fear of urban violence, the need for a slower-paced life, or opposition to the Vietnam War, Gerard J. O'Reilly of Detroit, who planned to join the American exodus, had still another reason. He was a medical defector.

A few years ago, leaving the United States was the furthest thought from Gerard O'Reilly's mind. He was a healthy and robust man of forty-two, earning $250 to $300 a week as a foreman at a Chrysler plant in Detroit and looking forward to buying his own home, perhaps even in the suburbs.

But in 1968 Mr. O'Reilly developed a chronic, serious,

and expensive kidney disease and began spending three days a week hooked to a kidney dialysis machine in Windsor, Ontario, because one wasn't available in Detroit. By March of 1971 he was unemployed, his family was living on the $100 a week his wife earned, and his health insurance was running out.

After Chrysler placed him on its permanently disabled list, Mr. O'Reilly tried to find another job. At first he was optimistic. State employment counselors changed his mind. "All these guys could do," Mr. O'Reilly remembered, "was sit down and look very profound and ask me what *I* had done. I got nowhere with them. They were the ones who were supposed to know the people. All I wanted was the connections. I was trying to help myself, but I couldn't even get that from them." One man tried to help because a member of his own family had a kidney disease. "I can still hear him," Mr. O'Reilly said. "His exact words were, 'If it wasn't for that, your case would have been taken and buried in the back drawer in a file and you would have heard nothing about it.'"

He continued to go from office to office and agency to agency. Nothing was available. The economy was off and most of Detroit had a "deep freeze" on hiring. He thought about going into the franchising business and negotiated with Dairy Queen for about a year, but that fell through, too.

As for his health insurance, Mr. O'Reilly used up the basic 365 days of hospital care in July of 1970. His major medical picked up 80 percent of the cost after that, leaving him with $140 a month to pay out of his own pocket.

But in June of 1973 Chrysler, which covers disabled workers for a period of time based on their length of service and the seriousness of their illness, would have made its last insurance payment on his behalf. At that point, Mr. O'Reilly would have found himself faced with an illness that costs $1,300 a month but without any insurance to pay for it; and no other Blue Cross policy that would have been open to him at that time included kidney dialysis treatment.

So he wasn't waiting. He was moving to Canada, where, for a total payment of only $309 a year, he, his wife, and their two teen-age daughters would be fully covered for all their hospital and medical care needs, including the cost of visits to doctors' offices.

The only limitation would be that the services be "medically necessary." Otherwise, the O'Reillys would be free of the clauses and restrictions that frequently plague many Americans who think they are fully covered against the cost of illness. There would be no limit on the number of days covered or the amount that could be paid out for any one person or illness. There would be no deductibles to pay before the insurance took over and no surprises when "extras" such as laboratory work and X rays were not covered.

"That means," said Mr. O'Reilly, "that every time I go to a doctor's office, every time I go to a hospital, every time I get a blood test, everything at all that is associated with medicine and hospitals is automatically taken care of."

He had some alternatives open to him in this country, but nothing that would carry him beyond the summer of 1973 and nothing that looked as good to him as the Canadian health insurance plan. For example, Mr. O'Reilly was eligible for some new kidney disease benefits that went into effect at Chrysler on April 1, 1971. They provided for immediate and unlimited kidney machine treatment on an outpatient basis, or for home treatment on a machine installed and paid for at no cost to the patient. If nothing else, this at least would have saved him the $140 a month that his major medical didn't cover, some $3,360 over the next two years. Yet even this had its drawbacks.

The outpatient care—available only in American hospitals—would have forced Mr. O'Reilly to find another doctor and leave the Canadian physicians who, he felt, literally saved his life and in whom he had absolute trust and confidence. In his mind, it was Canadian medicine, not American medicine, that kept him alive in the first place. He said kidney specialists in Detroit and his own doctor never explained how sick he really was when he first saw them in the spring of 1967. When he continued to feel tired and run down a year later, his wife, a Canadian citizen, suggested he see the Windsor kidney specialist who operated on her. "I wasn't in there three minutes before I went into the hospital," Mr. O'Reilly recalled. "In five days they told me the bad news. They were quite sure of it when they talked, and they impressed upon me the seriousness of my illness. I just couldn't leave the doctors in Windsor. They know me, my case, the whole history. They're my lifeline."

Why the outpatient care is good only in Detroit when Blue Cross of Michigan regularly extends its coverage to

Windsor is a mystery Mr. O'Reilly wasn't able to solve. All he knew was that he had been receiving outpatient care all along. But he was billed on an inpatient basis because that was the only way Blue Cross could make him eligible when he needed a machine in 1968 and couldn't find one in Detroit. Evidently, though, the rules only bend once. Having benefited by Blue Cross generosity and imagination in 1968, Mr. O'Reilly now felt victimized by Blue Cross bureaucracy and intransigence in 1971.

As for the home treatment, Mr. O'Reilly felt it would disrupt his family. One of his daughters fainted when she saw him being attached to the kidney machine in the hospital. Since his wife already worked eight hours a day in a factory and was under great pressure, he preferred not to put her through the additional strain of learning how to operate the machine so she could assist him with his treatments.

There was one way, though, that Mr. O'Reilly could have continued having Blue Cross pay the full cost of his Canadian treatment. If he went without any in-hospital services at all for 60 days, he would have been eligible for another 365 days. That wasn't 60 days of paying his own way, though. That was 60 days of nothing at all, regardless of whether he paid for it or not, for a man who couldn't live more than three days without being hooked up to the machine. Blue Cross people were as puzzled by this restriction as was Mr. O'Reilly. The only answer they seemed to have was that it might have been strange, but it was in the contract.

What Mr. O'Reilly needed, though, was not the chance to save some money on the cost of his treatment over the next couple of years, but some long-term security; and he needed it immediately. He couldn't afford to gamble that the next Chrysler health insurance contract would cover disabled workers on an unlimited basis for the rest of their lives, or that Blue Cross would change some of its rules to include him.

"I've got no real choice," he said. "I've got to go soon. I'm just an average guy. I didn't chase the buck that hard. I was content with the life I led. I raised my family properly and paid my dues to society, and all I know is that I got a kick in the tail for it. Now I've got to watch the buck and play the game the best I know so that it will be beneficial to me and my family. This is the thing I have to think about.

"I've got a total of about $8,000 in cash, stocks, and bonds. I'm not staying here and gradually watch my money dribble away bit by bit so that when I am absolutely and completely broke I can crawl on my hands and knees and ask people in this country what they are going to do for me now.

"But never in a thousand years will anyone ever be able to make me understand how a man can go through this in this country. It's almost obscene that an American should have to go to another country to get inexpensive medical care. When I go to Windsor they can't understand what has happened to me. All they have to do is pay their premiums and they get the care."

Not surprisingly, some Michigan Blue Cross people didn't see it that way. One was asked whether the technical distinction between outpatient services in the United States and inpatient care in Canada wasn't forcing Mr. O'Reilly to make some difficult personal choices in order to qualify for benefits that, though saving him a few thousand dollars, could easily leave him out in the cold at the end of two years. He replied that the O'Reilly case could also be viewed as a situation in which a man had rejected, for personal reasons, two alternatives that other kidney patients had found acceptable. "He is looking at this," said the Blue Cross official, "from the point of view that he will decide from his needs alone what he wants to have done. And of course health contracts are not provided in that manner, for the individual. If there were hundreds of people in his situation, we would probably change."

There *are* hundreds of people in Mr. O'Reilly's situation, probably even millions. They can be found in Michigan, Connecticut, and all the other forty-eight states. Not all of them have a serious kidney disease, and certainly leaving the country for medical reasons is a rare enough event. But that really doesn't make any difference. They are all living with exactly the same feelings Mr. O'Reilly has lived with—anxiety, uncertainty, and fear. And they want an end to it. They want more comprehensive insurance, and they want it made available in less complicated ways, feelings that are just as true for the family that has escaped unscathed as they are for the family that is $50,000 in debt.

Their reasoning is hard to beat: if other countries can

do this, why not the United States? Perhaps it is true, they agree, that no country in the world has had much success in controlling the cost of medical care, let alone reducing it. If anyone has, they have kept it a secret. But is that any reason why the United States should be alone among the major industrial nations in failing to protect its citizens against the high cost of this care? In America, where medical care is far more expensive than else-where, consumers still pay 37 percent of all medical bills, 39 percent of all doctor bills, and 13 percent of all hospi-tal bills above and beyond what their insurance covers, percentages that exceed anything consumers are paying in Canada, Britain, or Sweden. In some cases, certain figures for consumer spending don't even exist in other countries. The Canadian consumer price index, for in-stance, doesn't include hospital costs because the gov-ernment regards them as a public expense, not a per-sonal one to be paid directly or even partially by individuals.

No such luck in the United States. Medical care most definitely is a consumer item. Anyone who has ever tried to check out of a hospital only to learn there are some charges the insurance isn't going to cover can testify to that. So can anyone who needed medical care when he was beginning a new job in a new city, or was out of work, on strike, or waiting out the "qualifying" period insur-ance plans insist upon. Generally, people in these situa-tions aren't covered at all and have the choice of footing the bill themselves, or facing a collection agency, a law-suit by the hospital, or bankruptcy court.

Such events are not as infrequent as the country might

like to imagine. Whenever one occurs, it is a reminder that while medical insurance is supposed to be a form of protecting the patient, just as often it is an enormous gamble on the part of the patient. Because of restrictions and limitations individual insurance carriers place on policies, consumers invariably gamble that they won't succumb to certain illnesses, such as cancer, which requires therapy that is not fully covered in many plans; or kidney disease, tuberculosis, or mental illness, all conditions for which benefits vary greatly from plan to plan; or childhood diseases stemming from birth defects, which are rarely covered by anybody. The consumer must also gamble that he won't get sick at certain times, namely during the six-month to one-year waiting period various plans impose before declaring him eligible for benefits. And perhaps the biggest gamble of all is the gamble of those whose insurance pays only a flat and predetermined amount. They are gambling that the cost of medical care won't go up and that they will have no special problems or complications when they need medical care.

In Nashville, Tennessee, gambles like this are all that 90 percent of the labor union membership has ever known. Because the unions are small and can't negotiate for the cash to buy insurance that covers their members for the average daily cost of hospital care, they settle for indemnity insurance provided by commercial carriers as part of an accident, life, and health insurance package. So the 300 members of Plumbers Local No. 352 receive only $30 a day toward the cost of a hospital room that now averages about $46 a day. And they get that for only thirty-one days. Hospital extras, that catchall which includes laboratory work, X rays, drugs, special therapy, operating-room time, and intensive care, and which can knock the wind out of a family's budget and savings, are the patient's responsibility after the first $400.

The most any plumber can receive toward the cost of surgery is $250, an amount limited to 9 of the 147 surgical procedures covered by their health insurance plan, such as brain surgery or removal of spinal cord tumors. In maternity cases, everything above $200 must be paid by the subscriber. Last February a twenty-one-year-old apprentice took his wife to Vanderbilt University Hospital for the delivery of their first child, a boy. Complications developed, and although everything turned out all right, the family was presented with a bill for $1,160.85 —$960.85 more than the insurance paid.

When bills like this are added up, as the plumbers union did in 1969, they show that the plumbers are paying about $120,000 worth of hospital, doctor, and medical bills a year out of their own pockets—an average of about $400 a member. To James R. Krantz, union secretary-treasurer, that's money that could have provided a much better return for the members. "The out-of-pocket costs for health care by union members in middle Tennessee in the last ten years," he says, "could have established a prepaid group health plan covering all services." Had that occurred and the membership been able to pay a basic monthly fee for all their medical care needs instead of purchasing them item by item and illness by illness, then, says Mr. Krantz, people like George Hunt, fifty-eight, a retired plumber, wouldn't have had his $14,000 worth of savings wiped out in four years. "If a person saves up $14,000 over the years," says Mr. Krantz, "he should be able to retire without having to spend all his money for health care until he is penniless."

Between 1967 and 1969, Mr. Hunt had two severe heart attacks that forced him to retire. His medical bills came to $5,500. His insurance paid for $1,750, leaving him with $3,750 to pay back out of his savings, plus the 1-percent-a-month interest the hospital was charging him. Nevertheless, Mr. Hunt and his wife felt they were lucky—lucky to be still living in their own home (the mortgage insurance took over the payments); lucky that their five children were married and on their own; and lucky because Mrs. Hunt held back a little on paying the bills so she and her husband could stretch their retirement money a little longer.

That was how they felt in January of 1970. Later that month the roof began to cave in. Mr. Hunt underwent a prostate operation. Having used up all his hospital insurance on the heart attacks, he had a brand-new $2,000 hospital bill to pay. Coupled with the earlier $3,750 worth of medical bills, that brought the savings down to $8,250. Then he developed diabetes, which took another $2,250. He was down to only $6,000.

Living expenses began to mount and doctors' bills kept coming in to the tune of at least $800 a year, not including any X rays or electrocardiograms. The Social Security and pension money wasn't enough, and the

Hunts had to go to their savings. "The last time I looked," Mr. Hunt said in April of 1971, "I had $10 in my savings account and about $30 or $40 in the credit union." He also had a $700 hospital bill he hadn't paid off and he owed a doctor $150.

Individual consumers, though, are not the only victims of the cost of medical care. If medical costs continue rising faster than the cost of living, then some medical care programs may reach a financial breaking point, stranding whole groups of consumers.

At the rate medical costs are climbing in New York City, some 27,000 hotel workers and their families could be in this position fairly soon. The hotel workers have good, comprehensive medical care available at six family clinics, plus Blue Cross insurance for hospitalization. All the money to support the clinics and provide the Blue Cross coverage is paid by the employers. Ideally, all the clinics would have been hospital-based. But the Hotel and Motel Trades Council, the bargaining unit for the nine hotel workers unions, lost that battle to various hospital medical boards.

When the clinics opened in 1962, they had $9 million worth of reserves. Four years later, the clinics were in the red. By 1970 reserves had dropped to $5.5 million and the clinics were running a $625,000 deficit on their $3.4 million budget. It's the same story with the Blue Cross part of the plan. The union's insurance fund, which used to have a $1 million reserve for accident, sickness, and life insurance, in addition to hospitalization, is now flat broke. Everything could grind to a halt in another four or five years if the cost of operating both the medical centers and providing the Blue Cross coverage continues to outpace employer contributions by about 50 percent, as it has the past several years.

"Our plans are in real trouble," says a union official. "There's terrific pressure from the employers for the curtailment of benefits because of costs, to move away from Blue Cross, which makes you a captive of inflation because you're always paying the increase the hospitals pass on to them, and into an indemnity plan which everyone knows can only hurt our people. Hell, our average salary is only $100 a week. How can you pay part of the daily hospital bill out of that?"

Meanwhile, there are still stories of personal hardship in the hotel workers union. There always are. No matter how good the coverage is supposed to be, somebody always gets trapped

Luciano Velez, fifty, a kitchen worker, is one who did. His wife, a diabetic, was hospitalized for forty-nine days in late 1969 and early 1970. The bill was $5,895.95. Blue Cross paid $4,599.20. The "catastrophic illness" section of the New York State Medicaid program covered $310.63. That left Mr. Velez, who takes home $84 a week, with $986.12 to pay himself. The hospital wanted $300 down and $25 a month. He didn't have the $300 so he offered $20 a month instead. The hospital refused. He took his problem to the union and Mrs. Shirley Kronberg, director of the Neighborhood Service Councils of the Hotel and Motel Trades Council, negotiated with the hospital. They agreed to take the $20 a month.

"It is going to take him four years to pay off that bill,"

Mrs. Kronberg fumes. "And that's all he was trying to do anyway. He just wants to comply. He isn't trying to cheat anybody. But there is a whole superstructure and industry that is built on collecting medical bills from poor people."

Similarly, a printer in the Southwest, who prefers to remain anonymous, finished paying off a $40,000 bill in 1970 for expenses incurred during the thirteen months his daughter was under treatment for a tumor. He had been making the payments for fifteen years, since 1956. Half the money went to family members who carried him through the financial crisis, and though they told him the cash was a gift, he felt obliged to repay it. When one of the hospitals he owed filed a lawsuit against him several years ago, the printer switched jobs every few weeks to avoid having his wages attached. He owed the hospital $250. It's the only part of the $40,000 he refused to pay back.

Reduced health coverage, though only a possibility for the New York hotel workers, is already in the wind for others. Confronted with underwriting losses of $600 million on health and accident policies at the end of 1970, many commercial insurance companies have all but admitted they are on the verge of switching from the standard reimbursement of the cost of medical care to indemnity insurance. One of them, the CNA Financing Corporation, has gone ahead and made this switch in the basic hospital and major medical insurance it offers to members of trade groups. Beginning June 1, 1971, it also planned to withdraw its major medical coverage on an across-the-board basis and replace it with the indemnity type.

"We came to the conclusion," said David G. Scott, executive vice-president of CNA, which writes $15 million in annual premiums on major medical policies, "that this kind of policy is impossible to provide on a profitable basis in today's fast-changing world. Rate increases aren't enough. The more you raise rates, the more you squeeze out the average risks and end up with the bad ones that will buy coverage at almost any cost." In 1970 CNA raised premiums for individual major medical policies from 50 to 100 percent.

All of the above is how medical care in America can look to a patient who is squeezed in the vise of rising hospital costs and limited coverage provided by an insurance "industry" that is fragmented into 75 Blue Cross, 72 Blue Shield, and almost 1,000 commercial companies, each offering a variety of different policies based on a host of special restrictions and limitations. Consequently, having good health insurance isn't simply a matter of just walking in off the street and receiving the complete, comprehensive, and standard package of benefits that everyone else receives at a cost that is consistent with your income, as Gerard O'Reilly can do when he moves to Canada; it's a matter of living in the "right" city, working for the "right" employer, or joining the "right" union. In the last analysis, these circumstances—accidents of fate, even—determine how well protected any individual family is against the cost of illness. As Dr. Rashi Fein, a Harvard Medical School health economist, has said, "Only a discreet and diplomatic observer would say the situation is confused. A less tactful person might simply say, 'It's a mess.' "

The "mess" has been a long time in the making and nearly everybody seems to have seen it coming. Since the early 1930s, public and private study groups have been warning the country about the consequences of this situation. As a matter of fact, some of the concerns of the 1932 Committee on the Costs of Medical Care, a self-created and voluntary agency financed by foundation money and staffed in part by government experts, are remarkably pertinent to today's problems.

"The costs of medical care in any one year," the committee said, "now fall very unevenly upon different families in the same income and population groups. The heart of the problem, therefore, is the equalizing of the financial impact of sickness.

"The individual family derives no comfort from the knowledge that the *average* [emphasis in original] cost of medical care is not excessive for families with the *average* income. . . . The unpredictable nature of sickness and the wide range of professional charges for nominally similar services render budgeting for medical care on an individual family basis impracticable. On the present fee-for-service basis, it is impossible for 99 per cent of the families to set aside any reasonable sum of money with positive assurance that that sum will purchase all needed medical care."

Hospital insurance was a particular concern of the committee. "Although fewer than ten per cent of the population are cared for in hospitals in any one year," the report went on, "hospital illnesses are so expensive that they consume 50 per cent of the total annual expenditures for all medical care. . . . Hospitalized illnesses . . . bear with special weight on person in the so-called 'middle classes,' who can ordinarily meet the costs of minor, brief or non-hospitalized illness, but who cannot pay much more."

Yet not until the late 1960s when the Congress began paying the hospital and doctor bills for the Medicare and Medicaid programs did the problems of the individual consumer finally strike a responsive chord in Washington. Up to that time, federal involvement was restricted to the limited purposes of providing medical care for certain groups for whom Washington felt some special obligation, such as servicemen, their families, veterans, merchant seamen, and American Indians. Other than that, it stayed out of the medical marketplace altogether. Like the issues of the supply and distribution of doctors, questions of cost and financing of medical care were private and personal matters that individuals were supposed to work out for themselves with their employers, their unions, their insurance carriers, their hospitals, and their doctors. In Washington's eyes, medical care had not yet been elevated to the status of a basic human right.

Many attempts to change this attitude were made, but they all fell short of the mark. The earliest was the National Health Bill that Senator Robert F. Wagner, Sr., Democrat of New York, introduced in 1939. Based on some sections of President Franklin D. Roosevelt's National Health Conference report the year before, it sought federal matching grants for state public health programs. Though in many respects an innocuous measure and facing, said *The New York Times*, "only minor opposition in the Congress," the Congress nonetheless decided, with an assist from the American Medical Association, that the country wasn't ready for this type of federal activity.

Four years later, in June of 1943, following a *Fortune* magazine poll that showed 74.3 percent of the people favored national health insurance, Senator Wagner joined with Senator James E. Murray, Democrat of Montana, and Representative John D. Dingell, Sr., Democrat of Michigan, to introduce the first of the Wagner-Murray-Dingell bills.

A much more ambitious bill than the 1939 measure, it called for comprehensive medical, hospital, dental, and nursing-home care for practically everybody in the country, with the care to be paid for out of a special fund of employer and employee contributions. If the limited Wagner bill was too much in 1939, then the all-encompassing Wagner-Murray-Dingell bill clearly was a political fantasy in 1943. That didn't trouble the sponsors. They were looking to the future. But fourteen years later, the Murray-Dingell bill (Senator Wagner resigned from office in 1949) was still being introduced in the Congress and dying in committee.

In the meantime, the proponents of national health insurance, deciding that something was better than nothing, narrowed their objectives and pushed only for medical insurance for the aged. Here was a group that everyone could agree deserved assistance. Not only did they succumb to illness more frequently, but millions were living on limited incomes. Besides, the price tag was much smaller—$230 million as of 1951, compared to the billions of dollars the full-scale insurance program would have cost.

Lowering the sights, both in terms of those covered and the dollars involved, didn't shorten the battle or make it any sweeter. Both sides waged it relentlessly until the Congress finally passed the bill in the summer of 1965 and President Lyndon B. Johnson flew to the Harry S Truman Memorial Library in Independence, Missouri, to sign the bill into law.

Though a chink in medicine's laissez-faire armor had at last been found and exploited, some of the excitement was short-lived. Every piece of legislation must pay its political price on the way to becoming a law. Medicare's price was spelled out in Section 1801, which read as follows:

> Nothing in this title shall be construed to authorize any federal officer or employee to exercise any supervision or control over the practice of medicine or the manner in which medical services are provided . . . or to exercise any supervision or control over the administration or operation of any such institution, agency or person.

In other words, the federal government could reimburse hospitals and doctors for their services, but it couldn't use that money to change the organization or the availability of those services; nor could it effect much control over costs. Washington, with its several-billion-dollar health budget, was as much a captive consumer as the individual citizen with a hundred-dollar medical bill.

Furthermore, Medicare coincided with some major developments that had been building throughout the postwar years and that all came together to affect dramatically the cost of medical services in the late 1960s. Among them were an increased demand for medical care on the part of the consumer, the emergence of the hospital as the central institution in modern medicine, hospital insurance that frequently paid for only the most expensive kind of care, new equipment and technology, better pay for hospital workers, and last but by no means least, inflation.

The dam burst. In 1965, Social Security Administration officials estimated that the hospital portion of Medicare would cost $3.1 billion in fiscal year 1970. It actually cost $5.8 billion. The 1965 estimate of hospital costs in 1990 was put at $8.8 billion. That's been revised to $16.8 billion. Payments to physicians soared even more, going from $623 million in fiscal 1967 to $1.2 *billion* in fiscal 1971.

Much of this increase may have been inevitable, for, as Dr. Ernest Saward, former medical director of the Kaiser Permanente Clinic in Portland, Oregon, has pointed out, "We took the highest-medical-risk groups, the elderly and the poor, combined them with the highest-cost ser-vice, the hospital, and then stood around open-mouthed at the results."

Regardless, the fact that the cost of the Medicare and Medicaid programs caught the federal government so flat-footed had some positive benefit. At least Washing-ton was getting a better picture of what life had been like during the forty years the American consumer had been wandering in the medical wilderness.

It was also becoming clear that providing the money to pay for medical services was perhaps the smallest part of the job and certainly the easiest. Major overhauls were needed. They were needed not just to protect people against the high cost of illness but to offer them alterna-tives to the fragmented and largely pay-as-you-go fee-for-service medical care most now receive. If the country was going to spend more than $80 billion on medical care in 1972, then perhaps it was time to think about getting more bang for the medical buck by developing new forms of organization and delivery. Paradoxically, the most frequently suggested alternative, the prepaid group practice plan, was exactly what the Committee on the Costs of Medical Care tried to get the country to adopt back in the year 1932.

After all is said and done, though, it's still the cost of medical care that frightens people the most. And even if they find a way out of their financial troubles, as did Robert H. Schutz of Albany, New York, a $250-a-week Associated Press photographer with eight children, the emotional scars stay with them.

Mr. Schutz' son Rick broke his neck in a diving accident two days before his high school class graduated in 1968. He spent the next twenty-eight months in and out of six different hospitals and rehabilitation centers in four cities and underwent surgery nine times. The total cost was $75,000. Then in the fall of 1969, Mr. Schutz himself suffered three heart attacks, which added another $5,000 to the family's medical bill. Insurance covered $30,000, including the heart attacks, and a lawsuit against the swimming pool manufacturer provided enough cash to pay off the balance on Rick's $75,000 worth of care.

Looking back on the whole experience, Mr. Schutz feels, and his doctor agrees, that the relentless pressure of medical bills piling up on top of each other was a basic cause of his heart attacks. "Sure I was fat and forty-three at the time," he says, "but the strain was unbelievable. Nobody can afford that kind of money. I don't care if Nelson Rockefeller, with all his money, had this happen in his family. They couldn't afford it if they had to continue on their own after the insurance. It is such an overbearing wipe-out for the average guy. It just eats away at you. It eats, pounds, erodes, etches, whatever you want to call it. It takes away from you, and each litttle piece that goes never comes back."

People like Mr. Schutz have received widespread attention because the details of their troubles are so staggering and so unique. Yet, basically, is there any real difference between the Schutz family and the thirty-one-year-old Long Island widow with three children who is so short of funds that last winter she didn't pay a $50 doctor bill for six months? A $50 bill may not have much drama connected with it—unless it's yours and you don't have the money to pay it. But it's worth remembering that, as this widow says, "You can drown just as easily in two feet of water as you can in a hundred."

IV

The Health Business

EARLY in 1972, the American health care industry, a loosely organized and often unrelated composite of some 7,000 hospitals, 300,000 physicians, 1,000 insurance carriers, hundreds of other health care institutions, numerous medical supply and drug companies, and close to 5 million employees, attained a moment in the sun it probably had never anticipated ten years earlier.

It became a bigger business in the United States than national defense. The magic number was $79 billion. And while some of the health care industry's "success" in overtaking defense was due to a leveling off of defense spending, its growth from a $27-billion-a-year industry in 1960 to a $79-billion-a-year industry by early 1972 was clearly a matter of its own doing.

Where it is going from there is anybody's guess. If the current estimates hold up and the industry continues to grow at the current rate, the national health bill will total $120 billion by 1975 and close to $200 billion by 1980.

Should that come to pass—and there isn't a shred of evidence it won't—then at the end of the decade health will command a greater percentage of the gross national product (9.8 percent) than the defense establishment enjoyed at the height of the Vietnam War (9.1 percent).

As usual, hospitals will lead the charge, laying claim to fifty cents of every dollar spent for health and medical care in 1980, as compared with the thirty-six cents they claimed for every dollar spent in 1968. Doctors and dentists will take twenty-seven cents of the 1980 health dollar, and the remaining twenty-three cents will be shared by drugs, appliances, nursing homes, research, construction, and other health services.

Measured on an individual basis, this means that each man, woman, and child in the country will be spending an average of $814 for health care in 1980, compared to the $280 they were spending in 1968. They will spend $398 for hospital care (it was $102 in 1968) and $157 for physicians' services ($57 in 1968).

And looked at in terms of individual institutions, it means, according to the American Hospital Association, that the cost of a day in the typical two-hundred-bed hospital, which was $92.32 in 1971, will climb to $153.68 in 1975 and hit a peak of $263.15 a day in 1980, with the larger teaching hospitals weighing in at considerably more. (Though these figures represent a daily average of all costs incurred by a hospital in the course of a year and therefore, according to the hospitals, can't really be compared to the basic room and board charge that shows up on a patient's bill, some 80 percent of this amount eventually finds its way back into the basic room and board charge.)

Whatever this might mean to doctors, hospitals, and other providers of medical care, to the consumer, the man who eventually must pay the bill, it is very much of a mixed blessing indeed. Perhaps, if he is lucky, all those extra dollars will translate themselves into the kinds of improvements in organization, financing, and delivery that will make medical care easier to find and more pleasant to receive than it often has been in the past.

But he is not betting on it. Because from where he sits, it looks much more like a case in which public funds and third-party insurance payments have spawned the civilian equivalent of the defense establishment. And no matter how strongly the providers of medical care insist that the analogy is spurious, that nobody can, in good conscience, compare what goes on inside a hospital with what happens in a weapons plant, or equate the work of a surgeon with the duties of a battlefield commander, the two industries still look very much alike to the consumer. Both have an apparently insatiable appetite for money and an enormously well developed talent for avoiding public accountability and controls.

Few cities have had this combination of consumer frustration and industry lack of accountability documented as vividly as has the city of Philadelphia. It began in 1958, when Francis R. Smith, then the state's insurance commissioner, held the country's first public hearings on a Blue Cross request for a rate increase. They lasted eighteen days, and in granting Philadelphia Blue Cross a smaller increase than it had sought, Commissioner Smith issued a statement that said in part:

> If present methods of hospital administration are continued, if present practices are not corrected, the Blue Cross plans will be applying year after year for additional rate increases . . . [and] the whole scheme of prepaid medical care through the Blue Cross system will be irreparably injured at the expense of millions of citizens of Pennsylvania, resulting in severe personal and financial hardship and suffering.

Thirteen years later, when another insurance commissioner, Herbert S. Denenberg, held public hearings on the largest rate increase ever requested by Philadelphia Blue Cross, all of Mr. Smith's predictions had come true. Blue Cross had indeed raised its rates every year, so that the family that had been paying $4.95 a month ($59.40 a year) for its coverage in 1958 was being asked to handle premiums of $37.50 a month ($450 a year) in March of 1971. And the hospital bed that cost $20.17 a day in 1958 was going for $73.73 thirteen years later. For some, the rise in the cost of hospital care has been even more dramatic. Mrs. Evelyn Benham testified at the hearings that she was hospitalized three times for foot surgery during a recent five-year period. Each time, she said, she stayed on the same floor, in the same building, and had the same operation. As a matter of fact, everything was the same—except the bills. These were some of her charges:

Item	1966	1968	1970
Room & Board (per day)	$30.00	$45.00	$88.00
Operating & Recovery Rooms	50.00	100.00	250.00
Pharmacy	5.90	25.25	56.85
Radiology	22.00	56.00	65.00
Medical & Surgical Supplies	2.00	8.50	34.00

Furthermore, the basic problems of hospital management that former insurance commissioner Smith felt had to be solved if hospital costs and Blue Cross rates were going to be controlled were still the major bones of contention. They included such items as ending the duplication of hospital facilities; curtailing abuses arising from unnecessary hospitalization; providing outpatient care for people who didn't have to be in the hospital; providing more facilities for long-term convalescent patients as a low-cost alternative to prolonged hospital stays; and a study of all hospital financial practices, especially hospital charges.

A 1971 witness whose testimony had much to say on these issues was Samuel H. Fried, a sixty-five-year-old laundromat owner. Mr. Fried spent a week in the hospital in the spring of 1970, being admitted on a Saturday morning and leaving the following Friday. He entered the hospital because his throat felt as if something had been stuck in it for several days. As he described his experiences, though, they amounted to an almost classic case of a hospital stay gone haywire, of various abuses, arrogances, and inefficiencies that patients usually feel they are helpless to control and that nobody else apparently cares to control for them. Mr. Fried's chronology of that hospital stay is as follows:

First Day: Nothing happened—at a cost of $60 a day.

Second Day: Nothing happened again—for another $60 a day.

Third Day: A doctor showed up, "spent about ten minutes, looked at my throat using a tongue depressor, and said he could see nothing." For that, Blue Shield paid the doctor $15, and the doctor sent Mr. Fried a bill for an additional $10.

Fourth Day: Because Mr. Fried was scheduled to go for a barium X ray at 8:30 or 9:00 A.M., he ate no breakfast. The radiologist, though, was also on the staff of another hospital and didn't even arrive until 11:00 A.M., so Mr. Fried never went to X ray until 12:45 P.M. Then he became sick to his stomach—a combination of hunger, tension, and the fact that he "just couldn't stand having a large glob of dry barium paste that looked like something you would plaster a wall with" being put in his mouth for him to swallow. He went back upstairs. Later in the afternoon, his family doctor came in and "ridiculed" Mr. Fried for his behavior, though he did promise Mr. Fried that tomorrow, when the procedure was repeated, he would have the X-ray technician thin out the barium and add some chocolate flavoring.

Fifth Day: The X ray was completed. Yet Mr. Fried, a

former medical corpsman who had tried to keep up a little with medical knowledge, thought the whole procedure was unnecessary. His understanding was that a barium X ray was used mostly for people suspected of having stomach ulcers. He had no stomach problems of any kind, no disorders, no pain, no lack of appetite, nothing.

Sixth Day: His family doctor came to see him again. "I complained about the unnecessary procedures and asked him to discharge me," Mr. Fried said. "He said he would first have to get a report from the X rays and would discharge me the next day."

Seventh Day: The family doctor never showed up. So Mr. Fried discharged himself.

That ended Mr. Fried's seven days in March. It also ended his relationship with that particular family doctor. The doctor decided Mr. Fried suffered from arthritis of the throat. Mr. Fried, whose throat has been fine ever since, felt it was probably nothing more than a piece of soda cracker that got stuck on the way down. But what really angered him was the fact that the doctor, who charged only $6 for an office visit and $10 for a house call, was charging $25 for each hospital visit because he could collect $15 from Blue Shield. And then, Mr. Fried said, "the icing on the cake" was picking up a newspaper a few days later and reading that the after-tax profits of holding companies that owned hospitals had increased 38 percent the year before while their tax rate was dropping.

Generally, hospitals have responded to this type of

criticism by arguing that such abuses are relatively rare, and that even if they were nonexistent, it wouldn't have much effect on hospital costs. They would still be high. On this point, the hospitals are right. Like it or not, hospital care is expensive. It can't be bought on the cheap, not anymore at least. And this is by no means an American phenomenon. In Sweden, which many American health planners feel is a model of health care organization and delivery, hospital costs, measured both according to per diem costs and as a percentage of total health spending, have increased faster than they have in the United States.

As for the reasons behind the costs, the hospitals say this has been explained many times over. In a sense, they are right on that one, too, because the hospital litany of what has pushed costs up is almost as familiar as the consumer's recital of how much more he has been paying.

The key to it all, according to the hospitals, is that hospital and medical care is a personal services industry. It requires people, lots of them. A full 70 to 75 percent of any hospital's operating budget goes for wages, salaries, and fringe benefits, the cost of supporting the people who provide the medical services and maintain the institution. Though it sounds simple enough, even so obvious as to be trivial, it has been a difficult idea to get across to the public.

"The fact that the patient may have seen only two, three, or ten employees doesn't mean that nobody else has done anything for him," explains Dr. Mark Freed-

man, former administrator at Beth Israel Hospital in
New York City. "Hospitals, unlike other industries, have
standby and hidden costs, people who are available
should the patient need them. It's like the army, where
the number of front-line troops always seems so shock-
ingly low compared with the number of support troops
you don't see. And as technology increases, it seems like
the number of front-line troops gets smaller.

"It used to be that half the space in a hospital was
devoted to patient service. Now the amount of space
directly related to patient care is 20 percent. If you want
to go back seventy-five years, it was 80 percent. An old
hospital was all beds. There were no laboratories, records were a sometime thing, the business office didn't
exist, and the X ray hadn't even been invented."

Then there is the matter of hospital wages. They were
shamefully low for many years. From 1947 to 1967, hospital workers weren't even protected by the federal mini-
mum-wage laws. So while others were getting a dollar an
hour, kitchen and laundry workers in New York hospitals
were receiving sixty-eight cents an hour, and in some
southern cities as little as fifty cents. Nonprofessional
hospital workers now receive $2.50 an hour in larger
institutions, close to what they would earn in other industries for the same kind of work. Their continued demands, say the hospitals, are going to push costs even
higher.

It's pretty much the same story with salaried employees, such as interns, residents, and nurses. Nationally, interns' salaries nearly tripled in nine years, going

from an average of $2,800 a year in 1962 to $8,000 a year in 1971. At the bigger metropolitan hospitals, such as Mount Sinai Hospital in Cleveland, interns were receiving $9,000 a year in 1970, with promises of more to come, because that was what the hospital felt it had to offer to stay competitive with New York, Boston, and Los Angeles. To those who complained that the hospital had gone from exploiting interns (they were paid $600 a year in 1950 at Mount Sinai) to overpaying them, the hospital's director, Sidney E. Lewine, responded by pointing out that an eighty-hour week at $9,000 a year averages out to about $2.16 an hour.

The average salaries of residents have shown almost as large a jump. They went from $3,300 in 1962 to $7,500 in 1971. Oddly enough, the average salary for interns is presently higher than that for residents. However, it is expected that this situation will soon be reversed

Nurses' salaries also are rising. The nurse who was paid $86.50 a week in 1963 was making $144 a week in 1969 before taxes and without overtime. Hardly sensational, but livable. More increases are on the way, with California setting the pace. Some 4,000 registered nurses in the San Francisco area are due for $195-a-month raises by January 1, 1973, according to a contract signed in May of 1971 by the California Nurses' Association and San Francisco hospitals. That will boost the starting salary from $720 a month to $915, and the top salary from $840 a month to $1,035 a month. And the first stage of the three-step increase was retroactive to January 1, 1971.

"Look at what that really means," says a hospital official. "How in the hell can a hospital go back and tell the people it treated between January and May that nurses cost more while you were here, only we just found out. You can't. So what happens? You saddle the patients you have with the extra cost."

The payroll practices of the 1950s and most of the 1960s, the hospitals now admit, were inexcusable and kept hospital costs unnaturally low for too long. But, they say, the public is feeling more than just the rightful demand of hospital employees for more adequate wages. It is also feeling the pressure of inflation, which hit all the service industries hard during the sixties.

Next on the hospitals' list of what has happened to their costs is equipment and technology. Not only has medical knowledge increased enormously since the end of World War II, but most of the developments have resulted in a whole range of new equipment that runs all the way from throw-away hypodermic needles that avoid infections to $250,000 linear accelerators used in cancer therapy.

Mr. Lewine of Cleveland's Mount Sinai Hospital testified before an Ohio Insurance Department hearing: "This is an important portion of our dilemma, because as a hospital chief executive, I am not ready to say to our medical staff, which demands a coronary care unit once the evidence is in that the coronary care unit saves lives, that they cannot have it. Indeed, my job is to come before the board of trustees of our voluntary hospital and say, 'Here is the evidence, here is the cost, here is where the money is going to come from, and this is the impact on our operating costs.' Our money to do this thing in terms of capital is usually voluntary contributions, and I don't think there is a person in this room who, sitting on a board of trustees of an institution, would deny the services of such a unit to its public if there was any way that it could be accomplished."

Much of the new equipment and technology has a cost-push impetus all its own. Coronary care units are generally run at an 80 percent occupancy rate compared to the 90 to 95 percent rate an efficient hospital shoots for with its other beds. That's only the beginning. Unlike most industries, where the purchase of new equipment reduces labor costs, exactly the opposite happens in hospitals. A coronary care unit requires a nursing staff that is twice as large and twice as skilled, and therefore twice as expensive, as a routine unit. "Most of us," says Mr. Lewine, "are able to operate average medical or surgical patient care units at about a fifty-fifty or sometimes three-to-two ratio of non-nurses to nurses, that is, practical nurses, nurses' aides, orderlies, ward secretaries, and the like. This cannot be done in a coronary care unit. Indeed, the ratio runs about three-to-one, three registered nurses to one practical nurse's aide, orderly, or ward clerk." The same holds true for other specialized services such as surgical intensive care units, where costs can run as high as $300 a day.

Though hospitals frequently try to raise private funds or use trust funds or endowment money to purchase the most sophisticated and expensive equipment, the cost of operating and maintaining the equipment, which can easily exceed the purchase price in a fairly short period of time, is borne by the individual patient through his insurance premiums. As often as not, though, a hospital can't find the outside money, so the patient also ends up shouldering the purchase price. If the money isn't available, a hospital can save up its depreciation allowance to buy equipment or allocate the purchase price in other reimbursable ways. And the bulk of a hospital's machinery and hardware, says one hospital administrator, is reimbursable anyway, equipment such as X-ray machines, anesthesia machines, and physical therapy devices. In addition, equipment costs are rising. The electrocardiograph that cost $850 in 1968 went for $1,050 in 1970. A single X-ray unit can cost $100,000 and, depending upon technological developments, be obsolete in a few years.

From there, it's a short step to the next reason hospitals give for the rapid increase in their costs: they are treating a different kind of patient. The name of the game in the 1970s is heart disease, hypertension, cancer, diabetes: chronic diseases that are complex in origin and require long-term treatment. Often the life that is saved by a miracle drug, a surgical breakthrough, or a technological development is also a life of further medical complications and astronomical hospital bills. For instance, the Hospital of the University of Pennsylvania admitted a thirty-three-year-old man with severe stomach ulcers caused by alcoholism in June of 1970. Part of his stomach was removed. After he was discharged, the wound began draining. He was readmitted for surgery a second time. While recovering from that operation, part of his lung closed down and he was transferred to an intensive care unit that was only two years old. His fever kept "spiking" to 106 degrees.

A third stomach operation was performed, and the ulcerated area and a hole discovered in the large intestine were both repaired. But after surgery he had difficulty breathing and developed pneumonia. Again he was transferred to the intensive care unit. Only this time his kidneys shut down, and he developed an infection in his blood, began to lose his eyesight, and showed signs of heart failure. In addition, he couldn't eat and was being kept alive by a system of intravenous feeding that does not require any oral supplements at all and that had been in use only three years. Without it, he would have died.

While this meant life to the patient, even though his recovery chances were exceedingly slim, it also meant a large unpaid bill for the hospital. As of March 1, 1971, the man's total bill came to $101,803.62. His insurance covered $26,618.96, leaving the hospital with an unpaid balance of $75,184.66. Every year, says the hospital, free care and bad debts result in losses that it must pass on to other patients in one way or another in order to break even.

Another large loss the Hospital of the University of Pennsylvania recently sustained involved an American construction worker injured in a South American automobile accident. As of June 11, 1971, he had spent almost three years in the hospital, most of it in a coma.

His total bill was $80,115.16. Legal problems involving his family and his former employer, whose hospital insurance plan went out of business when he did, have prevented the hospital from transferring this man to a less expensive facility. The case is also a dramatic illustration of what the cost of a day in the hospital can do to a medical bill. When the man was first admitted on April 13, 1968, the daily room and board charge was $52. Two years later, the rate was raised to $88 a day—an increase that has added $13,040 to his bill in a single year.

Outpatient and emergency care are other areas where losses frequently occur, particularly with regard to patients covered by state and city medical assistance programs. Philadelphia hospitals lost some $15.9 million providing emergency and outpatient services in 1970, according to Daniel E. Gay, president of the Delaware Valley Hospital Council. The state of Pennsylvania reimburses hospitals for only three patient visits a month and at the rate of only $4.00 a visit when the actual cost of providing the care is $17.34 a visit. The city of Philadelphia pays even less and in addition cut its contributions back $1 million in 1970.

Many other factors also enter into the cost picture, such as more full-time salaried physicians on hospital staffs; the effect of inflation on all the goods a hospital purchases, such as food, linen, and medical supplies; the larger administrative staffs needed to handle the paper work and bookkeeping required by Medicare, Medicaid, and other insurance programs; insurance plans that cover routine diagnostic or minor surgical procedures when they occur in the hospital but not when they are performed in a doctor's office; and more expensive liability and malpractice insurance. Yet, essentially, from the hospital's viewpoint, they all add up to the fact that the modern hospital is a fundamentally different institution than it was twenty years ago, constantly redefining its role and offering new services to the community.

As Anne R. Somers of the Princeton University Industrial Relations Section has said, "Of all present developments in the health care field, the emergence of the modern hospital has been the most dramatic and the most impressive example of the institutionalization of medical care. Within living memory, an age-old institution for the custodial care of the sick-poor has emerged as the center of the medical world—a vast complex of expensive buildings, specialized equipment and interdisciplinary skills brought together for inpatient and outpatient care, research, professional and general health education."

Thus, say the hospitals, they are steering a precarious course between the Scylla of public expectations and demands for superior medical care with all the trimmings and the Charybdis of economic weightlessness that is afflicting the whole country. They are operating on fairly tight budgets, living from hand to mouth in many cases because payments from insurance carriers can sometimes be two years late, and pressured on all sides by doctors, insurance companies, consumers, various levels of government, and employee unions. "It's not a business or a job I would go out of my way to recommend," says one hospital administrator.

Well and good. But answers like this are too broad, too vague, and too general. They are as easy to use in justifying an unnecessary expense as a necessary one. And as Francis R. Smith, the former insurance commissioner of Pennsylvania, said after listening to roughly the same kind of testimony at the 1971 Philadelphia Blue Cross rate hearings, "If you will excuse my modesty, I didn't hear anything new from the hospitals. Many times they didn't even appear to change the material they presented at my hearing and this one." Nor, said Mr. Smith, did anyone appear to have done much work toward solving the basic problems. "If anyone had," he said, "would we have the same problems we have today to such a large degree?"

The biggest problem, in Philadelphia and everywhere else, is the part of the cost story the hospitals *don't* talk about in public, the fact that much of their behavior can —and should—be described as philanthropic enterprise run wild.

"In this business," says Dr. Mark Freedman, the former hospital administrator, "everybody wants to become a medical center. If you're a 50-bed hospital, you want to become a 75-bed hospital. If they're a 75-bed institution, they want to build a new wing. If they have 150 beds, they start thinking about becoming a teaching hospital. Every hospital has taken the attitude that they are in pursuit of excellence and damn the cost, go ahead. Every hospital has taken the attitude that we've got to do everything for everybody. Every doctor and every trustee wants his hospital to be the best. It's not a bad goal if you can afford it. But how much is enough?"

And on it goes, with hardly anybody asking whether the community really needs the program the hospital undertakes, whether the hospital has any way of sustaining it financially over the long haul, or whether it's going to do as much for patient care as it does for institutional and personal prestige. Everybody just digs in and spends the money, expecting, as Dr. Freedman says, "that God and the government will provide." And if not them, then Blue Cross.

Ironically, money really isn't the problem. Commitment is. Because once a hospital bites the apple, it's out of Eden. And it can start with the best of intentions. If a widower whose wife died of leukemia leaves a hospital $50,000 to support leukemia research, and he leaves it for the use of an individual doctor, the hospital doesn't turn him down because three other hospitals are already doing leukemia research. It takes the money. Then the doctor uses that as seed money. He gets a couple of federal grants, and maybe one more from a private foundation. He buys equipment, hires a staff. There might even be money for new construction to house his project. Then things begin to change. Federal money dries up. Leukemia research isn't fashionable. The foundations decide they aren't going to renew the grant. So the hospital is left with a laboratory, a staff, and some equipment.

One way or another, these costs start finding their way

into a hospital's operating budget, even though Blue Cross plans frequently won't reimburse hospitals for research. But there are lots of ways of getting around that, particularly when, as one hospital comptroller says, his budget is so complicated that it takes six months to prepare and one month to explain.

A more commonplace example can be found in almost every large university-affiliated teaching hospital. Before the federal ax fell on fellowship and research funds, whole departments in medical schools were devoting 70 percent of their time to federally financed projects in research and education and 30 percent of their time to insurance-coverage-financed patient care. Now that the Washington pipeline has dried up, the hospital–medical school complexes are trying to see how much of the medical school's 70 percent, which includes working space and equipment as well as salaries, can be transferred to the hospital's 30 percent.

"So the nickels start falling on the backs of the patients," says Dr. Freedman. "Is the service to the patient improved? Yes. Is it improved dollar for dollar by the transfer of people and space from the research budget to the hospital budget? It couldn't be. It increased operating costs far beyond their previous levels. And the question we have to start answering is whether the efforts put into those facilities really were necessary or did they grow only because money was available."

Frequently, it's the latter. Hospitals, like any other big businesses, are fierce competitors. In the battle to attract more doctors and more patients, they place an enormous, if unstated, emphasis on prestige and public relations in which the equipment, the research, the new programs, and the medical specialists are the chrome of the institution.

The push can come from many different places: from an ambitious and aggressive surgeon who wants only the finest and most modern equipment money can buy and nothing else; from an entire medical department within a hospital; from the whole medical staff; from a prestigious group of physicians outside the hospital; or from the board of trustees. Regardless of the source, the results are the same. They are the sign to the outside world that the hospital is a superior institution, engaged in one of the noblest of human missions: saving lives. Which it is. The trouble is that with hospital costs rising four times faster than the cost of living and twice as fast as wages, the "saving lives" argument, which is usually invoked in behalf of any large expense, is beginning to sound distressingly similar to the Defense Department's perpetual warning that the Russians, the Cubans, and the Chinese are coming.

Undoubtedly lives are being saved. But there appears to be an awful lot of waste, inefficiency, and personal pride that the consumer is financing in the name of medical progress. In Seattle, Washington, to cite one instance, the General Accounting Office of the United States Government recently surveyed health planning and coordination. These were some of the GAO findings:

• The five open-heart surgery units in Seattle hospitals

gave the area the capacity to perform 1,092 open-heart operations a year. In 1969, they performed only 318, and even the hospital that was doing most of the work was searching for more patients.

• The city had seven cobalt machines, which cost about $95,000 each to install. Six were in hospitals (one hospital had two); one was in a doctor's private office. If used at peak efficiency, that's enough for 154 cobalt treatments a day. On the average, only 100 a day were given over a one-year period—65 percent of capacity.

• Among the twenty-one hospitals providing obstetrical services, the average occupancy rate was 53.4 percent for beds and 47.4 percent for bassinets. Seven hospitals had utilization rates under 40 percent, and one had an 8.2 percent utilization rate. Fourteen hospitals reported a total loss of $1 million on their obstetrics departments in one year.

• Some fifteen hospitals were performing neurosurgery in the Seattle area, with the facilities being used less frequently than the open-heart surgery equipment. One neurosurgeon told the GAO investigators that most neurosurgeons were associated with two or more hospitals and spent much of ther time traveling from hospital to hospital. He suggested centralizing neurosurgery in one or two hospitals but doubted that the other hospitals would go along because neurosurgery, despite its infrequent use, was a money-maker for them.

• Though the Washington State Department of Health said in a 1971 report that Seattle would need only 3,951 hospital beds in 1975, by 1970 the city already had 4,291 beds and planned to increase that to 4,900 by 1975, or about 950 beds more than the state said it would need. Meanwhile, occupancy rates were low, averaging about 70 percent between October 1, 1968, and September 30, 1969. Five of the twenty-seven hospitals in the area had occupancy rates below 60 percent. One said it was because of poor economic conditions in the area; another said both doctors and patients preferred the more modern facilities of other hospitals, and the other three didn't know why the utilization rate was so low.

A few instances like this and a hospital is past the point of no return. It's no longer a question of there not being a proper incentive to cut costs and operate more efficiently. Now it's a matter of being penalized if you do. Reducing the length of stay and ensuring that no unnecessary use is made of a hospital bed may be a fine idea when it comes to saving the community some money. But it's a lousy idea as far as hospital finances are concerned, particularly if, as is frequently the case, utilization rates are not as high as they should be.

"In order to keep your head above water, you have to keep every bed filled," says one hospital medical director. "What good can a utilization committee do when the whole economic drive and thrust of a hospital is to fill up every available bed? The only successful way to run is to run full. If we could empty 10 percent of the beds, we would bankrupt the place."

That doesn't mean the medical staff is instructed to keep people in the hospital longer than necessary or to shanghai them off the streets and into the wards. It frequently does mean, however, that little pressure is exerted to encourage doctors to move their patients out as fast as they might. And, as everyone connected with a hospital freely admits, the longer a person stays in the hospital, the better the institution's chances of breaking even or making a profit on his stay. It's the first few days, when tests are performed, that are the most expensive. After that, it can be fairly close to downhill all the way if complications don't set in.

Such situations exist for an exquisitely simple reason: every hospital is an entity unto itself, a virtual fortress. It makes all its own decisions and is responsible to nobody else, at least not in ways that count.

The organizations the public thought had some influence on the hospitals either claim they don't or really don't. Health planning bodies and state and local government agencies are powerless or controlled by the hospitals. At best, they only "suggest," "encourage," or "persuade." A few planning bodies take great pride in the fact that they must approve all hospital expenditures over $250,000, neglecting to add that a hospital can go on a fantastic binge and not come anywhere near spending $250,000 for any single item. The GAO sudy of Seattle found that if a proposed project were privately financed and met state construction standards, then the Washington State Department of Health had "no other alternative" than to approve the project "even though it believes that the project will create excess facilities." The GAO report also said that the Regional Health Planning Council, which is responsible for health facilities planning at the local level, had "no effective means of preventing overconstruction."

Frequently the federal government can do more harm than good. An organization that wants to build a hospital can, if it is turned down by the Hill-Burton hospital construction program, go further down the street and get a loan from the Small Business Administration or the Department of Housing and Urban Development without too much thought being given to whether the community needs the facility or whether there is enough medical and nursing personnel to staff the institution. And one of the nation's most glaring examples of overconstruction and duplication are two federally funded military hospitals in San Francisco that opened late in 1968 and early in 1969, one for the Army and one for the Navy. The GAO and private hospital planners recommended a joint facility. The services refused, saying separate institutions were important for purposes of morale and medical training. Failure to consolidate has cost the taxpayers some $10 million in construction costs and an additional $8.2 million in operating expenses.

Even if individual communities started making more effective and economical use of their hospital beds and medical facilities, that still leaves the issue of how to exercise some control over a hospital's operating expenses. In theory, that's the job of the various Blue Cross plans and all the commercial companies that collect the money that supports the hospitals. Obviously, it hasn't worked out that way. Their traditional role has been *not* to exert any influence on how the money is spent.

Nobody really expected more of the commercial companies. After all, they were profit-making organizations and made no bones about it. They never saw their mission in life as cracking down on hospitals when the cost of medical care began increasing faster than the cost of living. For them, controlling costs meant cutting down on their "losses," which was how the companies described the medical bills they paid in behalf of consumers. So they put the squeeze on the patients. They added or increased coinsurance and deductibles, forcing the individual policy holder either to receive less medical care or to pay a larger portion of the bill himself, and sometimes both. Alternatively, some companies reduced the scope of their benefits or adjusted policies so that the man who thought he had a policy that covered the full cost of hospital care found out he now had an indemnity policy that covered only a fixed, flat amount. Policies were also canceled outright.

More was expected of the nation's seventy-five Blue Cross organizations, though, largely because the Blues were tax-free, nonprofit corporations that regularly espoused a philosophy of "public service." But the Blues have always suffered from a severe case of divided loyalties. They have seen their role as one of serving two masters—the public, which needs hospital insurance, and the hospital, which needs a steady income. And no matter how much Blue Cross or anyone else insists that the needs of the hospitals and the needs of the patients are one and the same, they just are not.

Perhaps it was different in Dallas, Texas, in 1929,

when a group of schoolteachers gave birth to the Blues by agreeing to pay Baylor University Hospital $6 a year per person for up to twenty-one days of hospital care during the Depression. But eventually the hospitals began to wield the real power and muscle within the Blue Cross organizations. They were the real winners in any conflict between patients and providers, so much so that in 1959, some thirty years after the establishment of the Dallas plan, the then president of the American Hospital Association, in his inaugural address, warned Blue Cross plans generally against acting as the "defender of its subscribers against the hospital rather than as an agency for the prepayment of hospital care *as it is determined to be by the hospitals and doctors.*" (Italics added.)

That idea has not withered on the vine. If anything, it may have flourished. For it is not uncommon today for a hospital administrator to claim, as one in the Far West recently did, that "we own Blue Cross." Certainly the hospitals dominate the Blue Cross boards. And when the spirit moves them, they frequently can do what they please.

Occasionally, the hospitals overreach themselves. Just before Pennsylvania's insurance commissioner, Herbert S. Denenberg, held his hearings in March of 1971, Philadelphia hospitals voted out of office as their representatives on the Blue Cross board both the chairman and the treasurer of the Blue Cross board because they had been instrumental in negotiating sharp cuts in Blue Cross payments to hospitals the year before. It was the first time in the thirty-two-year history of Philadelphia Blue Cross that any member had been denied reelection. But a week later, after the press had picked up the story, the full board reelected its deposed chairman, and for the first time in Philadelphia Blue Cross history, the chairman of the board wasn't even a member of the board.

In an immediate sense, though, the important issue is the one Commissioner Denenberg raised when he asked Philadelphia Blue Cross whether there should be "continuous dissemination of information to the public" regarding average per diem costs and charges; in other words, how Blue Cross felt about providing the consumer with a detailed breakdown—in dollars and cents and item by item—that would show the *difference* between what it cost a hospital to provide a patient with a hospital bed and what it actually charged the patient.

That's a real hot potato within the hospital world, especially since some hospital officials privately admit that charges "bear little relation" to costs, that as much as half a patient's daily charge for room and board represents "extras" the hospital adds on to cover its losses.

Yet what accounts for a hospital having such expensive tastes in losses? And what of other reports that nonprofit hospitals actually show profits of several million dollars a year? If it's true, what happens to the profits? Are they used to reduce the cost of hospital care, or are they poured right back into new programs that result in more prestige for the hospital and higher costs for the consumer?

There's no way to find out. Because when Blue Cross responded to Commissioner Denenberg's question, it parroted the hospitals' reasons for not divulging this material in the first place.

"No," said Blue Cross. "We believe that any reports concerning per diem costs and per diem charges to hospitals should be made only to the professional public, [such as] hospitals, [the] medical community, and certain agencies related to the health care field. The general public is not in a position to evaluate [this information]."

Commissioner Denenberg also sounded out Blue Cross on a couple of other issues. He asked Blue Cross for its opinion about making public certain information about their contracts with hospitals that traditionally had been kept private. In responding, Blue Cross said, "We do not believe any responsible public purpose would be served by the indiscriminate release of the detailed information relating to salaries, other operating expenses and financial stability which hospitals are required to make available under cost reimbursement contracts."

And he asked for Blue Cross views about providing the public with information regarding hospital payments to radiologists, pathologists, and other hospital-based physicians. Again, the same kind of answer came back: "No. We believe public disclosure of payments to hospital-based specialists would serve no useful purpose and could be extremely unfair to any such physicians. . . . We believe it would not be equitable to single out this group of physicians for this kind of investigation when similar investigations and reports are not made of all other physicians."

There is more that needs to be known. Why is it that

in Philadelphia people stay in the hospital an average of two days longer than anywhere else in the country? Are they actually sicker and in greater need of medical care or are they frequently there for "teaching" purposes? It's a question somebody ought to answer, because Philadelphia has six medical schools, more than any other city, and nine of the larger hospitals either are controlled by the medical schools or are operated in conjunction with them. And patients in teaching hospitals, according to information presented at the Blue Cross hearing, have hospital stays that are 22 percent longer than patients in non-teaching hospitals.

In New York City, why should there be a $49-a-day difference in the charges of two community (non-teaching) hospitals of the same size and with roughly the same kinds of patients? One charges $55.32 per day and the other $104.01. Is it the food, the nursing service, the kinds of procedures one hospital undertakes that the other doesn't, equipment, salaries, what?

If hospitals and insurance carriers were being asked to deliver the moon, that would be one thing. But they're not. They are being asked only for information the public has a right to know, the kind of information that normally is available when tax dollars are at stake and government agencies or programs are involved. The same standards ought to apply to insurance carriers and hospitals. Though they are private institutions, their missions are no less public than that of any government agency, and many of them have the tax-free status to prove it.

In short, the country just cannot afford to let hospitals and insurance carriers travel down the road of private decisions and voluntary controls any longer. "If anything," says Dr. Rashi Fein, a Harvard Medical School health economist, "health is going to be worse than defense. The Pentagon has tried harder than anything we in health have tried to use contractual procedures to estimate costs. I'm not suggesting the Pentagon has done such a beautiful job. But in health, you can't even tell when it's a cost overrun. At least for the smaller things in defense, you get the feeling that there are specifications for a product and a bidding procedure. We haven't been able to specify what the product is that we want people to buy in health and we have no bidding procedures. And we ask them to pay whatever we determine the price will be *after* we have sold our services. So in some sense, we can be even less optimistic about health than we are about defense."

The prescription, then, is for some rigid standards of public accountability and fiscal disclosure. "The public understands things can be better," says Dr. Fein. "They know it is not inherent in the system that medical care must be inefficient or inequitable. But you go on like that until an organized entity, which is government, due to consumer pressure and because of the responsibility that government should have to allocate money wisely, says we will not continue to buy a product without intervening to see if the product is produced in as efficient a manner as possible, that we are going to worry not only about financing but about the delivery system as well."

There are signs that the Blues want this kind of authority lodged somewhere in government as much as anyone else. The New York Blue Cross plan, for instance, is strong in its support of the state's new prospective reimbursement ruling that requires that hospitals be paid according to fixed and prenegotiated budgets and not according to the traditional manner of being reimbursed for costs already incurred. The result of that change, says Blue Cross, is that daily hospital costs, which increased 19.2 percent in 1969, slowed down in 1970 and increased only 16.9 percent and were expected to increase only 13.5 percent in 1971. New York Blue Cross also gives hearty endorsement to the cost control law the state's legislature passed in 1969. Payments to hospitals by government agencies and Blue Cross plans, the law states, must be "reasonably related to the costs of efficient production of such services."

And in its testimony at the Denenberg hearings, Philadelphia Blue Cross argued that "if the protection of the public interest is to be expanded, then it must be through the establishment of specific involuntary controls over the costs which hospitals incur."

As far as the hospitals are concerned, though, the voluntary way is the only way. Yet when the Delaware Valley Hospital Council submitted a list of recommendations for improving medical care in the Greater Philadelphia area, that list did not, Commissioner Denenberg said, "include one suggestion about what the hospitals might do to economize or provide better care." The hospitals, he said, had "nothing to offer . . . except that they want more money and they want to be protected from malpractice litigation."

With friends like that, who needs enemies?

CHAPTER

V

From the Operating Room

to the Courtroom

ROBERT J., AN East Coast insurance broker, first noticed the pain late one spring. It was an "obnoxious" and "annoying" pain, he said, that started on the left side of his nose and went "almost up to the bridge." Usually it began in the afternoon, around two, three, or four o'clock, but after dinner and a good night's sleep, it was gone. "It lasted maybe three or four hours and then it went," Mr. J. explained.

The pain persisted, and a few weeks later Mr. J. went to the ear, nose, and throat specialist who treated his four young children. He received two prescriptions, had sinus X rays taken, and was asked to return in three days. But that night, shortly after he began taking the pills his doctor prescribed, Mr. J. noticed a swelling in his left

eyelid. He waited another twenty-four hours before calling the doctor.

"Do you know what's causing this?" Mr. J. asked.

"No, I don't."

"Shall I stop taking the pills?"

"No. Set your alarm clock tonight and take them
through the night every four hours. Come in and see me
tomorrow morning."

The next day, the doctor irrigated Mr. J.'s sinuses,
gave him some injections, and told him to telephone if
the swelling didn't go down by afternoon. It didn't, and
the doctor admitted Mr. J. to a hospital the same day so
he could receive antibiotics intravenously. That night,
the doctor visited Mr. J., told him the X rays showed a
bony tumor growing in his left front sinus cavity just
above his eye and behind the forehead bone, and said he
was calling in a surgical specialist. Mr. J. was transferred
to the surgeon's hospital, and on the morning of June 17,
1967, a Saturday, he was wheeled into the operating
room.

He emerged three hours later, blind in one eye, and
with the chip of a surgical chisel lodged above the other.
At the time, neither he nor his family was told what had
happened, and they didn't receive much information in
the days that followed. As a matter of fact, Mr. J. didn't
even learn about the broken chisel until nearly four
months after the operation. And when the surgeon filled
out the hospital discharge sheet, for complications he
wrote a single word: "None."

That wasn't the end. Mr. J's head- and eye-aches continued. They became so severe he was kept on constant

medication, was unable to sleep, had only limited use of his good eye, and could not return to work at all. Finally, in the winter of 1968, some six months after the operation, Mr. J., still under medication and unable to work, filed a lawsuit against the surgeon, his two assistants, and the hospital. He asked for $1 million in damages and, in a deposition taken shortly thereafter, he explained his side of the story.

"The first thing I remember after the surgery," Mr. J. said, "was my wife trying to hold me up in bed, and there was a nurse's aide holding a pan under my chin, saying, 'Spit it out, spit it out,' referring to the blood that was coming from my nose and was going into my mouth. Then I just blacked out and I don't remember anything until that night or the next day when they took the bandage off my left eye."

It was then Mr. J. realized he couldn't see out of the eye. He also felt an "excruciating" pain, "like a mule had kicked me right between the eyes." He said he asked the doctor about the loss of sight and the pain and was told the trouble was "just a little hemorrhage" that would "clear up in a couple days."

But the "little hemorrhage" didn't clear up. Not during the eight days he remained in the hospital and not after he went home. However, Mr. J. said he did receive the beginnings of an explanation from his doctor. A week after he was released from the hospital, he said the surgeon told him he had "nudged" the eyeball during surgery, but that the sight would return if Mr. J. would just "give it time."

Two weeks later, when his sight still hadn't improved,

he asked if the surgeon was "kidding," if his sight really would come back.

"It's got to come back," Mr. J. quoted the surgeon as telling him.

Mr. J. grew very apprehensive. For the next two months he tried to learn what might have happened during the operation. He began with the assistant surgeon. But he came away empty-handed. All the assistant would say, according to Mr. J., was that the eye was "just bruised a little bit" and that he didn't want to answer any more questions because "I had nothing to do with it."

Mr. J. also saw some ophthalmologists, particularly when, near the end of August, the hemorrhage behind the eye burst, turning the whole eye bloody red. He said one doctor told him he thought that in removing the growth "something pierced the eye or the ball" and "that's how the blood got in there" in the first place. He said another thought the eye had been "severely hit" during surgery.

In the meantime, the surgeon, who had been ill and on vacation most of the summer, returned. Mr. J. made an appointment for mid-September. "I just leveled with him," Mr. J. said, in describing their meeting.

"Was there an accident during surgery that caused the eye to be blind?" Mr. J. asked the surgeon.

"No. What makes you think that?"

"Look, I asked you what happened to the eye at one time. You said it was nudged a little bit. I asked Dr. ——— what happened to the eye. He said it was bruised a little bit. I asked Dr. ——— what happened to the eye. He said it looks like it was pierced. I went to another eye doctor. He said it looks like it was severely hit. What happened?"

No response.

A few more weeks passed. Mr. J. went back to the surgeon and told him he was losing confidence in the ophthalmologist the surgeon had recommended. Then "out of a clear blue sky,"said Mr. J., some four months after the operation, the surgeon told him about the broken chisel. As Mr. J. recalled it, the following conversation occurred:

"During surgery a chisel splintered," the surgeon said. "We have recovered all the splinters except one. It's nothing to worry about. It's just a little splinter." (He took out his pen and drew a small circle on a piece of paper.) "It's only about that size, it will flush out. There is nothing to worry about."

"Where is it?" Mr. J. asked. "Where is it located?"

"It's up here above the right eyebrow."

"How do you know—if it's such a small piece, how do you know you missed it? How do you know you got it out? How do you know you got all the splinters out?"

"We pieced back the chisel and we took an X ray."

Mr. J. kept pressing for details in subsequent visits. "I kept asking him to tell me the truth as to what occurred," he said. "He admitted to the accident but as far as any details were concerned, he wouldn't discuss it. I tried to find out what the heck took place, what was going on in there, and he just refused to say anything. I'd go in and he'd just hang his head. He kept saying [my sight] would come back. He kept telling me, 'Give it time.' "

Meanwhile, another eye specialist told Mr. J. the eye was hopelessly lost. This new specialist also ordered X rays, which revealed the chisel chip near the right eye. But, said Mr. J., "it wasn't just a round speck that was going to flush out. It was a quarter of an inch square."

More of Mr. J's side of the story was contained in a second pretrial statement, this one given by the physician who served as Mr. J.'s medical expert. It was his "conjecture" that when the chisel splintered, the "ricocheting effect of a piece of metal may well have pierced the left eyeball."

But essentially, Mr. J.'s medical expert was concerned with much more fundamental issues. From his review of the medical records and all the statements given in pretrial depositions, it seemed that the surgery itself was "premature," having been performed on the basis of an "essentially . . . inadequate" diagnosis and examination. Furthermore, he said, "It would appear that Mr. J. had little time to think about the advice of the consultation surgeon . . . [and] that he was immediately whisked away into the hospital. He did not have time to think over what was going on."

He also questioned whether the surgeon had the proper qualifications and skills to perform the operation, or had in fact been operating in a medical field that was beyond his training and competence.

The medical expert suggested the latter might have been the case, because an osteoma (the medical term for Mr. J.'s tumor) is one of those borderline medical problems that can fall within the domain of a neurosurgeon, an ophthalmologist, or an otolaryngologist (ear, nose, and throat). The surgeon in question was the latter. But in the absence of a "more adequate" preoperative evaluation, the expert said, it was impossible to say which of the three specialists would have been better qualified. All he could say was that if an "appropriate" neurosurgical technique had been used—such as the "cranial route" through the top of the head—then "chiseling might have been avoided and the osteoma taken out in mass" and "much of [the] subsequent damage . . . may well have [been] avoided" as well. But regardless of the technique used, said the physician, the operation was clearly one in which "an ophthalmologist or a neurosurgeon should have been in on the operation to begin with." None was.

The case came to trial in the fall of 1970, and, after several weeks of testimony, Mr. J.'s attorney accepted the defense offer of a $300,000 settlement in exchange for a signed statement that payment of this sum would in no way be considered an admission of guilt or negligence by either the physician or the hospital.

Because, in the mind of the surgeon and the hospital, there had been no negligence. Their side of the story, as related by the surgeon's attorney, was that the surgeon most definitely was qualified to perform that particular operation, even without consulting a neurosurgeon or an ophthalmologist. The defense's medical experts testified to this. They also said the cranial route suggested by Mr. J.'s medical expert would have been far more dangerous than the forehead procedure that had been used, so dangerous that just using it might be considered evidence of malpractice.

What happened, said the attorney, was an accident; an accident with tragic consequences, but an accident just the same, the kind of human error that nobody can predict or prevent. At the time of the operation, according to the attorney, the surgeon did not know Mr. J.'s eye had been injured . So it was natural for him to expect that the loss of sight that developed was only temporary. Nor, said the attorney, did the surgeon tell Mr. J. he had "nudged" the eyeball during surgery. What probably happened, the attorney speculated, was that eye retractors used during the operation caused enough pressure on the globe of the eye to alter the globe's location, because there was "no question that the location of the globe was altered," and this, apparently, had caused the loss of sight. But, he repeated, such damage was not known at the time of surgery.

As for the broken chisel, the attorney said that the surgeon had indeed failed to tell Mr. J. about this until four months after the operation. There were two reasons, said the attorney. First, the surgeon felt Mr. J. was suffering great pain and emotional stress following the surgery, so he decided not to say anything until his patient was feeling better. Second, the surgeon became ill a month after the operation, was away for two months, and therefore really didn't have the opportunity to inform Mr. J. until much later than he might have wished. But medically speaking, the surgeon felt the chisel chip had nothing to do with the fact that Mr. J. couldn't see out of his left eye and continued to experience severe and prolonged head- and eye-aches months after the surgery. The chip wasn't imbedded in his skull or any portion of his head or face; it was just "loose in the right frontal sinus cavity," said the attorney, and, in the opinion of his client, not causing Mr. J. any trouble whatsoever.

Finally, said the attorney, one had to consider the fact that the operation may have saved Mr. J.'s life. "When you have drainage blocked up from a frontal sinus," he said, "and when you have infectious fluid accumulating behind it, it has nowhere to go. Eventually, it will break out somewhere, usually in the brain, so that you can wind up with a brain abscess and meningitis. This tumor he had slowly and inexorably was filling his frontal sinuses. It wasn't going to be a life-threatening situation in the next twenty-four hours; but in the next week, three weeks, or six weeks, something had to be done to get that tumor out of there."

To the hospital, this last point was the key issue in the whole case. "The doctor saved his life," the institution's chief executive officer said in response to a question about whether any thought had been given to reprimanding, sanctioning, or disciplining the surgeon. "The tumor was the largest the doctor had ever seen. In removing it, apparently some vessel of some sort was ruptured or hemorrhaged that caused the blindess. But it was either blindness or death. We are talking about an extremely capable man, fully certified, and on a medical school faculty, highly qualified.

III

"The patient took advantage of the situation. He got $200,000 probably, after the lawyer took his share, which may be twenty times what he would have made in his entire life. And it was all tax-free. The problem in malpractice cases such as this one is that trial juries are all composed of laymen who are sympathetic and empathetic to patients. And if there is any evidence of incapacitation of the patient after treatment, they will vote to support him. But really, it is very difficult for anyone not connected with medicine to adequately judge these issues."

And that was the end of the case. Because unless somebody files a formal written complaint against a doctor either with the county medical society or with the state board of medical examiners—neither organization feels it has the necessary legal authority to review any individual case on its own initiative, no matter how serious it appears to be—then nothing more happens.

Some time after the case was settled, however, the doctor did apply to the county medical society for malpractice insurance. His application was accepted. The review committee felt he was a highly competent surgeon who often undertook some of the most difficult cases in his field. Since no disciplinary action was brought, the reviewing committee concerned itself only with his insurability.

But suppose, for the sake of argument, disciplinary action had been brought. Suppose the medical society decided there wasn't a shadow of a doubt on any of the issues; that the doctor knew Mr. J.'s eye was permanently damaged; that there wasn't a reason in the world to justify waiting four months before explaining the broken chisel; that he rushed his patient into surgery without adequate medical evaluation; and that he was operating in a field beyond his surgical knowledge and ability.

What then?

Would his license to practice medicine be revoked, suspended, or restricted? Would he be reprimanded or placed on some sort of probation? Not very likely. The annals of malpractice are virtually barren of examples in which physicians have been disciplined following a case. "To my knowledge in the state of California," says David M. Harney, a prominent Los Angeles negligence attorney, writing in my Senate subcommittee's 1969 report on malpractice,[1] "no physician sued for or guilty of medical malpractice has ever been disciplined by reason thereof." His views are echoed by Dr. Martin L. Norton, a Detroit anesthesiologist who is also an attorney: "There is no doubt in my mind that not a single physician has ever lost his license or even been reprimanded by a medical society based on his involvement in malpractice or on the incidence of malpractice cases in which he was involved."

Although medical malpractice suits and negligence actions have been increasing rapidly during the past sev-

---

1. Senate Subcommittee on Executive Reorganization and Government Research, "Medical Malpractice: The Patient Versus the Physician."

eral years, they still are not a particularly reliable way of assessing the overall quality of medical care generally rendered by America's physicians and hospitals or the ability of medicine to police its own ranks. There just are too few cases from which to make an informed judgment, and too many situations in which the facts, though they lean heavily in one direction, are never fully resolved.

But for the moment at least, a malpractice suit is the only vehicle a patient has, and the courtroom is his only public forum, for engaging the medical profession in a dialogue about the quality of care rendered in a particular instance, and thus for attempting to hold doctors and hospitals accountable to certain basic standards.

There's a lot wrong with this process. It occurs after the fact. It seeks to achieve what many feel are two completely separate goals—financial compensation for an injured patient and improvements in the quality of medical care. And the truly important issues are often lost in the personal bitterness that characterizes negligence suits in general and medical malpractice actions in particular.

Yet, since there are no public review boards of any kind, or public participation in medicine's self-policing efforts, it's all that exists; and it's one reason why malpractice suits, once so rare that insurance companies waged a vigorous campaign for the business of doctors and hospitals, have now become so prevalent that many insurance companies are dropping out of business altogether. (The increasing number of claims, the higher investigative costs, and the larger amounts paid out in settlements and verdicts have made malpractice a losing business, and therefore an unattractive one, say the insurance dropouts. Those companies that still write malpractice insurance, like Aetna Life & Casualty, say they are feeling the pressure almost as much. In the four-year period between 1965 and 1968, Aetna's underwriting losses for both doctors and hospitals, on a nationwide basis, went from $300,000 a year to $9.5 *million* a year.)

But a patient's feelings that he is unable to exercise any control over the quality of care he receives short of filing a malpractice suit certainly isn't the reason doctors prefer to talk about when they gather to discuss the malpractice "epidemic." To them, the growth of malpractice is the result of a wholly different set of factors.

The first is that the entire nation seems to have gone suit-crazy, and that doctors, like everyone else, have come in for their share of this phenomenon. As Dr. Michael J. Halberstam, a Washington, D.C., internist, wrote in his article on the subject in *The New York Times Magazine* of February 14, 1971:

> The peasant morality has just about disappeared from this nation. Misfortune is neither inevitable nor the will of God. If something bad happens, someone, some human agency, is at fault. . . . If the housewife finds a roach in her baking soda, if your best friend stumbles over the patio curb in your backyard, if one car hits another, out come the lawyers. The primacy of the automobile in our way of life has conditioned us to friend suing friend, the common effort to re-

build one's car after a slight accident, and to going to court for injuries that our horse-riding
ancestors would have rapidly (albeit painfully)
shrugged off. If a man is no longer reluctant to
sue his best friend (after all, the friend's insured),
he has no reason to refrain from suing his doctor
(who's also insured).

The second is that a combination of increased specialization by physicians and a much more mobile and no-
madic population as a whole have made medicine more
impersonal. Anesthesiologists, for example, are "easy
targets" for lawsuits. It's partly because they control life-
and-death situations and partly because nobody ever
thinks in terms of "the friendly family anesthesiologist."
"The anesthesiologist," Dr. Halberstam wrote, "in-
troduces himself the day before surgery, does his job,
sees the patient in the recovery room and, God willing,
never again." With regard to the changing population
patterns, malpractice suits seem to be much higher in
places like California where people are less likely to stay
in one place long enough to develop close personal relationships with their doctors.

There's also the doctor shortage, which the American
Medical Association says has increased the possibility of
the kind of breakdown in the doctor-patient relationship
that can lead to a lawsuit. Its effect on malpractice, as
analyzed by the AMA in a statement prepared for my
Senate subcommittee's malpractice report, is the following:

The average patient load and the average volume of units of patient care for the average physician has increased dramatically in the last five to six years. Medicare, Medicaid and the increased coverage of medical and hospital insurance have produced a skyrocketing rise in effective demand for medical services. Since the supply of physicians could not be increased proportionately, the demand could be met only by the existing number of physicians providing more units of patient care. . . .

Higher volume of patient care inevitably produces a higher exposure of legal risks and a higher volume of suits.

And finally, doctors feel victimized to some extent by certain aspects of the legal system. What troubles them most is the way trial attorneys are paid. They work on a contingency fee system, earning nothing if they lose a case but anywhere from 25 to 50 percent of the award if the case is won or settled. A system like that, the doctors contend, produces precious little incentive for a trial attorney to assess a case strictly on its merits before taking action. On the contrary, it's practically an engraved invitation for him to file suit whenever he feels there is the slightest chance he can convince a jury his client suffered unnecessary harm, pain, or injury.

"The doctors I defend," says Los Angeles attorney H. Gilbert Jones, "have no objection to an injured patient receiving financial compensation. What they object to is that in order for this to happen the doctor must be brought to trial and stigmatized. And believe me, that's a stigma, even if the plaintiff's attorney goes to great pains to tell the jury the doctor himself is not on trial and that the only issue is how much physical and emotional suffering his client underwent."

Dr. Halberstam has encountered the same situation. A physician who had been sued told him, "Goddam it, I took care of her for twenty years, saved her life twice, and she's suing me. Told me it wasn't personal, that she knew it wasn't my fault, that she still liked me. Wasn't personal! I'd hate to see what she considers really personal. I haven't been able to sleep right since my lawyer told me about it."

Any of the reasons doctors give for the increase in malpractice suits are true enough. And nobody can honestly doubt that this is a desperately serious problem for doctors, or ignore the fear of physicians that they will be sued not because they are negligent, nasty, or thoughtless, but because they are not perfect; because, like everyone else, they are human beings who make mistakes in judgment and who sometimes are just plain unlucky. It's the medical version of Monday-morning quarterbacking, say the doctors. A patient's condition may look unbelievably simple three months after the fact, when the full diagnosis has been made and the patient has taken a turn for the worse. But it's a far different situation for the doctor on the firing line during the early days of treatment.

Similarly, one cannot discount the effect that malpractice suits have had in forcing doctors to practice what they call "defensive" medicine. They refuse to treat some patients and order excessive and perhaps unnecessary tests and procedures for others. Though it drives up the cost of medical care, hopefully it keeps the lawyers at bay. "I was sued once because I didn't order a full set of X rays for a patient who really didn't need them and certainly couldn't afford them," says a California orthopedic surgeon. "Never again. From now on, every patient who I even vaguely suspect might conceivably need X rays gets the full set whether he can afford it or not and even if I don't really believe he needs them from a medical viewpoint. It's the only way I can stay in business and keep my malpractice insurance down."

But on the other hand, a strong case can be made that doctors were unrealistic in expecting that, in the absence of any other method of accountability, patients would not eventually resort to the lawsuit; unrealistic in assuming, as many have and still do, that one should no more think of suing one's doctor than one should think of suing one's clergyman, that it was both improper and immoral to sue a "good" doctor, generally defined as someone with the right credentials about whom seldom was heard a discouraging word.

In addition, those doctors who feel malpractice cases are mostly flukes and accidents, having no wider lessons for medicine as a whole, may be doing both themselves and the public a major disservice. "You should know," says Dr. Milton Alper, anesthesiologist-in-chief at the Boston Hospital for Women, "that the increase in malpractice suits has stimulated concern and interest on the part of some physicians about what it all means in terms of our social responsibility. In my own field of anesthesiology, it appears that the incidence of death or major disability as the result of an anesthetic mishap is low as compared to the number of people who need and get anesthetic care for surgery or obstetrics. Should we therefore view each such event as a fluke, a built-in, unavoidable, though statistically rare hazard of anesthesia? Or would it be more productive to take another attitude?

"Many of us believe that for every such tragedy, there may be many more instances where the potential for such an outcome exists as the result of corner-cutting, inadequately qualified personnel giving anesthesia, lower standards for obstetric anesthesia than for surgical anesthesia, etc. The adoption of the latter attitude and the collection of data to prove or disprove it would, in my opinion, be of much more potential benefit to the public."

Finally, a convincing case can be made that doctors didn't stay out of court ten or fifteen years ago because they were more careful or practiced a superior brand of medicine. There is probably more caution exercised today and better medicine being practiced. Doctors stayed out of court because they were reluctant to testify against each other—the so-called conspiracy of silence—and because the courts held doctors accountable only to local standards of medicine—the "locality rule." National standards were not recognized. If a physician from Massachusetts testified in Missouri that, in his opinion, the Missouri doctor had been negligent and there were more than enough journals, medical meetings, and other means for the Missouri doctor to have known the error of his ways, that didn't mean very much. What counted was the kind of care a patient could reasonably expect to receive in Missouri or in the particular community in which the alleged malpractice occurred.

Around the early 1960s, the locality rule began to crumble. But it wasn't until 1965 that any court, in this case the Supreme Court of Illinois, found a hospital negligent for not meeting even its *own* standards of medical care. In that instance, a central issue was what obligation state licensing regulations, national accreditation standards, and a hospital's own bylaws imposed upon an institution. Were these criteria meaningful or just window dressing? Did a hospital have to measure up to them or could it scale down its performance and responsibility to a lower level whenever problems developed?

Even after this decision, it took another two years before the Supreme Court of Washington broke legal ground by stating that "negligence cannot be excused on the grounds that others in the same locality practice the same kind of negligence."

In these respects, what is astonishing about malpractice is not how many suits may have been filed in recent years, but how late the concept of public accountability has been in coming to medicine. This is even more apparent when one looks at the various laws and mechanisms that exist to protect the public from poor medicine, or the possibility of it, and that organized medicine has developed, had a hand in developing, or could exert a major influence in changing.

State licensing laws are a good example.

Though medical knowledge has increased four hundred times in the past twenty-five years, licenses are good for life. They have no limitations. A general practitioner can perform brain surgery if nobody cares enough to check out his credentials—or forgets. As for relicensing, that is just a formality. It takes a signature, a fee, and nothing else. Only in New Mexico are physicians required to submit evidence of professional growth in order to maintain a license to practice medicine.

The California legislature has tried to follow suit. In March of 1970, it considered a bill requiring proof of continuing education at four-year intervals, one year later than New Mexico requires. But the California Medical Association obtained a three-year delay. The state's physicians said they needed that time to develop some extensive programs in continuing education.

Only four state medical societies make continuing education a condition of membership: the Oregon Medical Association, the Pennsylvania Medical Society, the Arizona Medical Association, Inc., and the Massachusetts Medical Society. The first two didn't take this action until 1970; Arizona and Massachusetts followed suit in 1971.

In addition, the effectiveness of the licensing examination itself is open to question. There is a complete lack of consistency about passing grades and considerable doubt about the qualifications of many examiners. And, says Dr. Robert C. Derbyshire, a past president of the Federation of State Medical Boards, state medical societies and boards keep waiting to make sure "the political climate is right" before rewriting "even the most hopelessly antiquated" licensing and medical practice laws. That moment, he points out, "never seems to arrive."

So the country limps along with what Dr. Derbyshire, in his book *Medical Licensure and Discipline in the United States,* called the "veritable patchwork of definitions . . . and standards" that are the sum total of the various state laws regarding the licensing and practice of medicine. There is such a wide divergence, Dr. Derbyshire wrote, that "anyone studying the statutes . . . will wonder how any state can accept the certificate of another. . . .

"The staunch advocates of states' rights," he went on, "defend the situation by saying that every state has its own peculiar problem and that the medical practice laws have been written with these in mind. But is this really a defensible position? Is the science of medicine so inexact that uniform standards cannot be applied throughout the entire country? Is there such divergence in the practice of medicine throughout the states that it must be governed by such a variety of laws? In the current age of the jet plane and easy communication parochialism is unjustifiable."

The result is that "every now and then," as they say in the medical profession, a case slips through such as this one described by the medical director of a 250-bed hospital in the Midwest:

We had an intern who was number two in his class at a major medical school. He was a native of the area. We actively sought him. After two months, though, it was evident something was wrong. He was setting fractures without a resident or a staff physician supervising. It was clear he resented all supervision and he was beginning to do stuff he wasn't trained to do. We called him in and told him he was taking responsibility beyond his education. He said it didn't matter because he was going to Africa to become another Schweitzer. He had a country all picked out and he had written a constitution for its people.

We decided he was a paranoid schizophrenic and we paid for some psychiatric testing and examinations. Three psychiatrists agreed that he was psychotic. We brought him in, showed him the staff reports and the tests and told him he could stay on but he had to receive psychiatric care. He refused and he threatened to sue, but when his lawyers saw what we had they agreed there wan't a case. So he leaves. And the next I hear he is in another state and has a license to practice medicine because they have no internship requirement. Then, through reciprocity, he switches to a state that wouldn't have let him have a license in the first place and he's practicing in a small town that has given him all kinds of honors. The last time I saw him he was in worse shape than before. If both he and the town are lucky, nothing bad will happen. But if it does, you can bet it'll be written off as God's will, an act of fate.

But the whole point is that it is virtually impossible to stop a graduate of a medical college from getting a license and practicing medicine if he hasn't committed a crime. One way or another, he'll find a loophole or a state law that fits what he wants and then use the licensing system to his advantage.

And what do the various state laws have to say about taking legal action against an individual doctor? They are clear enough about violations regarding narcotics, alcoholism, abortions, and felony convictions. But they are vague and even nonexistent when it comes to a physician's competence, his ability to practice medicine.

According to the most recent data available (published in 1965), in thirty-two states the law does not even mention professional incompetence as a reason for suspending, restricting, or revoking a doctor's license. The bylaws of thirty-eight state medical societies do not list professional incompetence as a basis for formal action against their members. And the states that have written incompetence into the law generally offer only elusive concepts. What does it mean to be "habitually incompetent," or guilty of "gross negligence," or exhibit "unprofessional conduct"? How many patients is that—one, five, ten, twenty, forty? Does the question of incompetence apply only in cases of outright venality and callousness, or does it include well-intentioned but questionable treatment as well? And according to whose standards?

There is some legal merit to these ambiguities. They protect the individual doctor against arbitrary attempts to revoke his license or judgment on the basis of a single bad result. They grant him due process and the right to remain innocent until proven guilty. But the other side of the coin is who is defining and defending the rights of patients? For a doctor can cause considerable harm or unnecessary pain and suffering and still not come anywhere near breaking the law. A world of difference exists between the legal definition of professional incompetence and the medical definition. And while it is natural for society to hesitate before restricting a man's ability to make a living, what happens when the legal case cannot be made against a doctor whom even other doctors regard as a hazard? Does he continue to practice? In most states, that is frequently what happens and why it generally seems that the law does a far better job of protecting the rights of doctors than the rights of patients.

"Sometimes," says the chief of medicine of a 350-bed hospital in New England, who has had his problems getting action out of his state medical board, "the best we can do is shift the risk from those patients who are in the hospital to those patients who are not. We can protect ourselves from a lawsuit, but we can't protect the community from poor medicine." His principal battle with the state medical authorities had occurred a couple of years before and involved a physician who had been dropped from the hospital staff some fifteen years earlier. (The hospital felt the doctor had improperly treated a broken leg and had engaged in questionable practices with regard to his fee. The hospital filed a complaint, and the state medical board reprimanded the doctor for "fraudulent, dishonorable, and unprofessional conduct.")

"I just happened to be in the emergency room early one morning around 2 A.M. when a woman was rushed in by ambulance," the chief of medicine said. "She was almost dead from heart failure due to rheumatic heart disease. All of that could have been corrected by appropriate medicine and eventually you could begin some repair with cardiac surgery. But here was this same doctor. He was treating her in her own home by applying paper towels soaked in camphor oil on her legs and chest.

"She had with her a grocery bag full of symptom medicine, tranquilizers, aspirin, cough medicine, nothing really specific, which the patient was instructed to take, was taking, and was proceeding to die. We took care of this patient and I reported the doctor to the state health department. They investigated, all right. They sent field interviewers to see me and many other doctors in the community who had come across this doctor's activity through problems in other patients. But nothing happened. The doctor still is practicing medicine."

The reason? One case wasn't enough to charge a man with "incompetence," "habitual negligence," "unprofessional conduct," or any other violation listed in the state's medical practice act, according to the state health director: "The attorney general said anybody can make one mistake, but you need more than one to act under state law." And, said the health director, himself a doctor, the state's hands were tied with regard to obtaining evidence of any additional examples of poor medicine practiced by the doctor in question. "By law," he explained, "a doctor can refuse you access to his records. It's easier to investigate if he is on a hospital staff, because those records are simpler to come by. But this man wasn't on any hospital staff, so we would have had to go through the files in his own office. We weren't sure what we were looking for, and you just can't enter a doctor's office and go on a hunting expedition."

So the next time the chief of medicine was confronted with medicine he felt was a risk to the community—he was involved in such instances in each of the next two years—he took no formal action at all, except to participate in a hospital decision to drop the doctor from its staff.

The first concerned a general practitioner who had been misdiagnosing cases, prescribing inadequate medication for patients suffering from heart failure and stroke, and generally practicing a careless and possibly even negligent brand of medicine. He was placed under strict supervision on the theory that keeping him on the staff where he could be watched was better protection for the public than turning him loose. But it didn't work out. Though the doctor notified other physicians when he admitted patients to the hospital as instructed, he didn't follow the medical recommendations of the supervisory physicians. In fact, he countermanded them. At that point, the hospital's executive committee decided it had no alternative but to completely rescind the doctor's hospital privileges.

The second involved a pediatrician who also was unwilling to accept any kind of advisory supervision after the hospital had reviewed his records and presented him with what it felt was evidence of poor patient care. In the medical staff's judgment, the doctor was administering too many intravenous fluids. It was also deeply concerned that the doctor had given exchange transfusions to three infants who may not have needed them at all, or at least not at that time. (An exchange transfusion is a gradual process by which the infected or damaged blood supply is withdrawn and a totally fresh supply fed in.) The pediatrician had the same problem at two other hospitals in the community, and the net result was that all three hospitals dropped him from the staff.

"Maybe I was wrong not to report these other two doctors," the chief of medicine said sometime later. "At least there was more than one case to go on. But at the time it just seemed to me that if they didn't act in that first situation, which was so outrageous and such an open-and-shut case, they just weren't going to act. Period."

But whether he was right or wrong isn't the point. The real issue is why he even had to make that decision in the first place: why, when a doctor is dropped from a hospital staff, isn't there some sort of automatic review procedure at the state level, just as a matter of professional ethics and public trust? Surely that would be superior to the present system of placing the entire burden for a more general review of a disciplined physician's competence on the back of a single doctor; in short, making the whole process dependent upon one person's judgment as to the merits of the case and the mood of the board.

Yet, by and large, questions like this have a very short history within the medical profession itself, let alone as public issues. All too often, medicine has just shrugged off discussions of the quality of medical care, the competence of physicians, the effectiveness of self-policing efforts, and the importance of public accountability by claiming that most doctors were honest, conscientious men who were trying their best to do a good job, and that the problems came from "a few bad eggs," just as in any other profession. Maybe so. But that sounds distressingly similar to an airline posting a sign above its ticket office saying, "Ninety-five percent of our pilots know how to fly." Furthermore, as Dr. Lawrence L. Weed of the University of Vermont Medical School has said, "When we start peddling honesty and thoughtfulness, we're bankrupt. The patient should get that for nothing."

Instead, what ought to be peddled are (1) a national licensing and medical practice law to bring uniformity to the chaos that now exists in this field; (2) more rigorous and widespread efforts at continuing education; and (3) local systems of quality control and self-policing that avoid the two flaws plaguing most of medicine's efforts in this area.

The first is that quality control and self-policing mechanisms are too limited in scope. They come to a grinding halt the moment a problem doctor is out the hospital door. After that, he is on his own—and so is the public. He can stay in practice, because he doesn't need hospital privileges for that. He can join the staff of a small, unaccredited hospital. Perhaps he will decide to obtain a loan from the bank or a federal agency such as the Small Business Administration and build his own hospital. He can move to another city or another state. So while he may be out of sight and out of mind to the hospital and the medical staff that originally discharged him, he is very much a clear and present danger to others.

The second is that the whole system is much too personal in nature. If one doctor doesn't stand up and point an accusing finger at another, nothing at all may happen. And pointing the finger isn't as easy as it sounds. Not only must a doctor make sure his case is sound, he must decide whether he is willing to put himself through the meat grinder of calling a fellow physician to task: overcoming the there-but-for-the-grace-of-God-go-I syndrome, and being fully confident nobody will find in his own medical records some quirk with which to return the favor. Very soon, he may be reconsidering, deciding that Dr. Jones is really a pretty good guy after all: his patients like him, he hasn't hurt anybody so far, he's the source of more than a few referrals, their wives play bridge, if he's really a serious problem how come nobody else has noticed, and everything probably will work out all right in the long run.

A very human reaction. But also symptomatic of a

hospital with a poorly developed system, or no system at all, for sifting out its potentially serious problems before they become personal disasters or lawsuits.

"I have gone through dozens and dozens of hospital bylaws," says Dr. K. J. Williams, director of medical affairs for the Catholic Hospital Association, who has evaluated medical practice for both Catholic and non-Catholic hospitals, "expecting to find some provision by which the administrator or the chief of staff has the official authority to suspend a man immediately when patient safety is at stake. And you seldom find a provision whereby they can do this in a current case. You have to wait until the end of the month to have an executive committee meeting. That's not good enough. All hell can break loose by the end of the month.

"After twenty years of looking at these kinds of problems," says Dr. Williams, "I am convinced that by and large most community general hospitals don't have the real quality control. They don't have the framework to minimize the incompetence and to do something about it. They have controls for some gross things, and many hospitals are extremely conscientious about protecting the public through critical self-analysis or peer review. But in this business, in which the stakes are life and death, you should be going to the fullest extent possible to minimize incompetence and establish good quality control mechanisms."

Life can get much more sticky than that. Dr. Williams says he has much more contact than he would like to have with situations in which individual physicians or hospital administrators want to do the right thing but are left completely out in the open with no political support or assistance at all. He has, he says, experienced instances recently in which:

• A local medical school refused a hospital administrator's request for a board-certified specialist to review and render a judgment on the skills of a surgeon who, it was suspected, may have been responsible for the deaths of two patients.

• A national specialty board (some have suggested these boards are the key to controlling quality and establishing national standards) turned down a request to provide an outside assessment of a doctor's competence. The board said if any of their consultants went into the hospital for this purpose, he might be sued by the doctor in question.

• A hospital administrator who did not want to grant temporary privileges to a young physician before checking his credentials finally caved in when he stood alone against the press, the local clergymen, and the three most influential physicians on the hospital staff. It later developed that the competence of the doctor in question had been criticized twice in the hospital he had just left and that none of its fifty staff physicians, or the administrator, was willing to provide him with a set of references or recommend him in any way. "The young physician," Dr. Williams said, "solved the hospital's crisis by, in the midst of all the fuss, quietly folding his tent and going south a couple of hundred miles to another hospital, another hospital owned and operated by the *same* religious order."

For Dr. Williams, the lesson of all this is that medicine is far too important to be left to the doctors. Since hospital boards are legally responsible for the quality of care that is rendered in their institutions, thanks to a 1957 court decision, it is up to them to demand that doctors use all the methods and tools available for assessing whether the quality of their care is as high as they would like to believe. That also means some drastic improvements in the mechanisms for finding, controlling, and disciplining incompetent doctors. This may be a very tough pill for doctors to swallow. They're not used to this kind of accountability. But the courts are calling for it, and so is the public.

Who knows? It may even reduce the number of malpractice suits.

CHAPTER

VI

The Long, Winding Road

to Medical Reform

IT TAKES NO special wisdom to see that many of the problems the American people face in finding and financing medical care are due in large measure to the fact that this country does not now have, and never has had, a national policy on health and medical care. Or at least not a policy that represented any clear, specific, and positive statement about the medical care that the citizens of this country were entitled to receive, and the financial and social conditions in which they were entitled to receive it.

This is neither an accident nor an oversight. Except in special circumstances, federal activity was looked upon as unnecessary. If we would just have faith in the competitive pressures of the marketplace, and the natural laws of supply and demand, everything would sort itself out in a matter of time. Doctors would practice where the need was greatest, and they would enter those specialties that people needed the most. Health insurance would be available at reasonable prices and would include a generous range of benefits. The actual practice of medicine itself would be organized in a manner that was mutually acceptable to both doctors and patients. Finally, the cost of medical care would stay on an even keel with the rest of the economy.

And by and large, the American patient would be the chief beneficiary of this natural ebb and flow. As the person who needed the service, the person for whom the system was supposed to exist, he would automatically become the center of the medical marketplace, the controlling force, the one individual who could set the tone and the tempo of the whole arrangement. He could pick and choose what he wanted, use his purchasing power to force the providers of care to be competitive and courteous, and, if he were dissatisfied, take his business elsewhere. That was how we had arranged for the distribution of every other kind of good and service in this country, so why shouldn't it work out just the same for medical care?

The truth of the matter is that it did. And that's precisely the problem. Because the American marketplace, as presently constituted, has always done much more for providers than it has for consumers, worked far better for the people who had something to sell than for those who were looking for something to buy. By any standard —price, availability, accessibility, convenience, accountability—consumers have invariably come out on the short end. And while that may be something we think we can tolerate as far as automobiles, refrigerators, and television sets are concerned, it clearly is not something we can tolerate where medical care is concerned.

For medical care is not like any other product. People don't purchase it on a whim, on happenstance, or in accordance with the latest styles. Few people, a very few indeed, play keeping-up-with-the-Joneses when it comes to medical care. Nobody goes charging off to the hospital to have open-heart surgery, a kidney transplant, or a hernia operation because they are the "in" procedures this year, the diseases the jet set has made fashionable from the coast of California to the Côte d'Azur. The man with a ruptured appendix or the parent whose child has a high fever and convulsions at four in the morning is hardly in a position to go shopping around for the best hospital bargain in town or to insist that he wants only that amount of treatment which is covered in his health insurance policy. He goes where his doctor tells him and he accepts the treatment he needs. Or if he doesn't have a doctor, he goes to the closest emergency room.

Furthermore, the person who needs routine medical services is in much the same position. He is a captive consumer. He obviously cannot go without medical care. Yet he is virtually powerless to influence or alter the medical care system in any meaningful way. All the major decisions and decision-makers are out of his reach, beyond accountability. There is virtually nobody of any consequence acting in his behalf. The American system of medical care is strictly a providers' system. They designed it, they built it, and they run it. They decide who will be treated, where they will be treated, when they will be treated, and how they will be treated. They decide how much each service will cost and how much will be covered by insurance. And they stubbornly resist any outside controls, on the theory that they are honest men of high moral purpose.

The trouble with that kind of arrangement is not that it leads to graft or corruption, that most doctors are stealing patients blind, or that hospitals regularly turn people away from their doors because they don't feel like working today.

As a profession, American medicine has a sense of responsibility and a code of ethical standards that surpass anything found in law and politics. The flaw is that such a one-sided marketplace, one so totally devoid of any significant consumer or governmental influence, invariably leads to an inbred kind of thinking. It becomes a marketplace in which the providers of care often fail to understand, and really have no incentive to understand, where their privileges end and the rights of patients begin.

"The rights of patients." We have bandied that phrase around so often and so casually in this country that it often seems little more than a cliché, a phrase to be trotted out when everything else fails, the conversation-stopper of the medical care debate. Be that as it may, the concept of the rights of patients is really what the current effort at medical reform is all about. It is the one thought that distinguishes the 1970s from the other major periods of medical change. Thus the early 1900s focused on medical school reform, on eliminating the fly-by-night schools, the phony degrees, and the quackery that passed under the name of medicine. The post–World War II period stressed medical research and scientific developments, the conquest of disease, and the development of new technology and new therapy. It was the period of the physician as scientist. And now, at last, in the 1970s, our concern is not the medical school, though we want to improve them; not the support of major research, though we do not want to abandon that; but support of the individual patient.

More specifically, our efforts are an attempt to establish as clearly as possible the following proposition: to receive medical care is the right; to provide it, the privilege. In a fundamental sense, that is really the only issue in medicine. That is all medicine has ever been about, or should have been about. That is all it should ever be about. Unless this country can accept the undiluted truth of this statement and make it the basis for national policy and national action, we are likely to face a much more severe version of what we have come to call "the health care crisis" for the rest of this century and well into the next.

Describing a problem is one thing, recommending a solution quite another; and the transition between the two is often an unsettling and humbling experience at best. For it is always much easier to describe what is wrong than to try to figure out how to correct it, to philosophize about the nature of the solution than to come up with the solution itself, to emphasize the need for change than to understand what ought to be changed and how it ought to be changed.

If, for example, the medical marketplace is flawed, and if, as seems entirely likely, the country decides that the health of its people is much too essential a natural resource to be left so completely to the private marketplace, we will have to decide whether the marketplace is flawed beyond repair or whether it can be improved by regulation and controls. And if the latter is the case, what kind of regulation and controls? That is an easy question to ask, a very difficult one to answer.

Similarly, the idea that we want to establish a more open and equal relationship between doctors and patients is a worthy objective, one many physicians and medical educators not only agree with but can articulate far better than the rest of us. "I don't know how it happens," a medical school dean once remarked to me. "Maybe we train it into them in medical school. But doctors, more than any other group of people, refuse to admit to their own self-interest. They think every decision they make is made for altruistic reasons, for the benefit of society or the individual patient, when the truth is that most of their decisions, or at least a good portion of them, are made because of what is most convenient and comfortable for them. That happens everywhere, not just in America. It's a worldwide pattern. And you have to see this day after day to understand how deeply imbedded this is in the medical school personality, imbedded in an archaeological sense so that you really have to dig and scrape around for years just to find it, let alone try to root it out or alter that kind of thinking.

"It is so deep, transmitted in so many subtle ways, that the doctor often cannot help but see himself as some sort of modern-day saint. In his own mind, he is a totally selfless person who is curing the sick and the afflicted. He means well, he is highly motivated, and when you get beneath the commercial sheen that's on the surface you can find a pretty solid streak of idealism and service. But many doctors seem constitutionally unable to accept criticism from outside the profession, or even to engage in an honest and open intellectual debate about the kinds of authority [a doctor's] training qualifies him to exercise, and the kind of authority it does not qualify him to exercise."

That is a provocative statement, a fascinating insight. Yet the man who passed it on to me would be, and was, the first to admit that while he knew what it was he wanted to change, he didn't have any clear idea of how he could change it, or how anyone else might.

He knew in general. He wanted to bring more non-medical people onto his faculty and to get his students out in the community to see what medicine was like from the patient's point of view. He hoped that the federal government, since it was already picking up a large share of the costs of medical education, would be more specific about the kinds of doctors it wanted medical schools to

produce. He also felt that consumers ought to participate more in the decisions affecting the medical care they
received, and that, if rebuffed by the providers, they
ought to demand to participate, even to the point of
filing lawsuits if necessary.

Yet while he felt strongly about each of these ideas,
and while he felt they were eminently worth trying to
work out on their own, regardless of whether he could
measure the success of any one, he kept insisting that
they still weren't much more than ideas, suggestions
really. They weren't programs, all fleshed out and ready
to go. They were skeleton outlines at best.

He was right. That was all they were because that was
all they could be. The frustration he felt in this particular
instance is the frustration that is matched a thousand
times over when we confront the entire spectrum of
problems affecting the medical care the American people
receive. For though we would like to have a program to
match the depth of our feelings, to be able to end some
of the more flagrant inequities, abuses, and absurdities
immediately, we are in the agonizing position of being
only on the fringes of the whole medical care issue. We
have barely begun to regard it with the seriousness it
deserves. We have just awakened to our responsibility as
a nation, and we are learning that while it is simple
enough to say that everyone should have the right to
receive care quickly and conveniently, that they should
have the right not to worry about how it will be paid for,
and they should have the right to be treated with dignity
and respect, ensuring those rights or devising the pro-

grams that seem most likely to ensure them is a complex and awesome task.

I say this not to discourage any particular recommendation or movement toward reform, not to put down a good idea because it is not yet fully developed, and not as an excuse for avoiding the kinds of major legislative actions we ought to make within the next two or three years. I say this because for the past several years I have been deeply troubled by the tendency of those of us who are the country's political leaders to behave as if every idea we offered were a full-blown program; and as if every program, no matter how limited the information upon which it was based, were a complete and total solution; so that if the country would just follow us down the glory road, we would reach the Promised Land, Shangri-la, or wherever it was we were supposed to be headed, by the day after tomorrow, or by next Thursday afternoon at the latest.

This has been one of the most disturbing trends in American politics. Why it has persisted for so long is not really clear. One reason seems to be that it permits politicians to take ego trips whenever we feel the need. We find a problem, proclaim a need, work up a five-point solution that takes fifty seconds to explain, make a speech, bask in the applause, and trundle off in search of new worlds to conquer, and then, shortly afterward, wonder why the problem still exists. Just as the doctor seems to be incapable of accepting his own self-interest, so we politicians seem incapable of admitting our own fallibility and our own limitations.

We seem unwilling to admit the truth about legislation, that it is only speculation: a theory, a hope, a guess, a leap of faith. All we are saying in any bill is that we think this proposal is worth a try. This is the program that represents the best of our collective thinking, or what we hope is our best, about the step the nation needs to take at this point in time.

But because we do not do this, because we are not honest with ourselves or with the country, because we feel that if we tell the truth we won't have the support that we need, we oversell most programs we pass. The result is obvious. Nothing lives up to expectation. Everything is viewed as a failure. Perhaps even the most carefully conceived, generously funded, and honestly explained program would be judged in this manner. For our sense of social consciousness is not as generous as we like to think.

Yet basically, our problem seems to be that we expect solving social problems will be like manufacturing automobiles or sending a man to the moon and back. Social change is not the assembly line writ large. It is not a matter of laying out all the parts and putting them together as the conveyor belts move our way, so that, at the end, we see exactly the product we expected to see, and it works just as we expected it to work.

Social change is much more complicated. And the lesson we need to learn is that rarely do we get the kind of "comprehensive" results we always say we are after, that shiny new package with the chrome and trimmings. More often than not, we settle for something less, because, in the first place, that is the nature of the political process, and, in the second place, that's how social change comes about. It comes in bits and pieces, pushes and shoves, nudges and bumps, through what the sociologists call "marginal" change.

That means social change requires a political maturity we evidently do not have and a staying power we wish we didn't have to have. It means there is no end to the process of solving social problems. They always continue to exist, sometimes in their old context, sometimes in a new one. For a nation that is impatient to keep its date with destiny, that is a hard fact to accept. But at this point in our history, we might be far better off to worry less about that date with destiny and concentrate more on our rendezvous with reality.

But where do we start?

We really don't have much choice. We start with financing problems, the national health insurance question. That is the issue that pushed medical care off the back burner to begin with and turned it into a topic of national importance.

In one sense, we are lucky. At least a dozen different bills were introduced in the Congress during the past few years dealing with various methods of financing medical care, or portions of it. They included bills that originated with such organizations as the American Medical Association and the Health Insurance Association of America, the insurance industry's spokesman.

It is easy to discount these developments as nothing more than special interests trying to block important reforms. It's more than easy. It's downright tempting.

But as somebody who went through the Medicare battle with the AMA in the early 1960s, who listened to and often was the brunt of some of the more hysterical and vitriolic comments put forth by that organization and its members, it is refreshing to see them at least propose a program, even though it is the weakest of the lot (it provides for tax credits for the purchase of health insurance by the affluent and purchase by the government of private health insurance for the poor).

What's more, one of the better ideas for reforming American medical care has come not from government, not from any radical reformer, not from liberals in the House and Senate, but from the American Hospital Association. It calls for the establishment of health care corporations that would be directly responsible for the health of a specific population group. Though its financing mechanism is a complex, Rube Goldberg type of arrangement, and though it carves out for the hospitals of America a much more dominant and autonomous role than we might like them to have, the idea, which builds on the success of the prepaid group practices, is one we cannot afford to pass up. We may not yet know how to make medicine directly responsible for the health of individuals. But it is the kind of objective we ought to pursue with all our energies.

There are also bills introduced by President Nixon and Senator Edward M. Kennedy. The Nixon bill would establish a system of national health insurance setting federal standards for the private health insurance purchased on the open market. The Kennedy bill proposes a national health insurance system that is both financed and administered entirely by the federal government.

In the current economic climate, there is a certain attractiveness about the Nixon proposal, or any other that focuses on shoring up the existing insurance system and using federal dollars to cover those areas where the need appears greatest. They call for less public spending and obviously would create the least disruption to our traditional arrangements and institutions.

Another idea with immediate appeal is to hold everything in limbo for a while and settle for something less than national health insurance, like a package that included coverage for catastrophic illness, improvements in Medicare and Medicaid, and perhaps something in the field of child and maternal health.

But if we want to make medical care a right in this country, a right in fact as well as in principle—and that is what our goal ought to be—then we have only one choice. We must move as quickly as possible toward a federally financed program of national health insurance. The program should establish a system of universal entitlement, one program for the entire nation. It should be open to everyone without exception and have no restrictions on the medical services that are covered or the length of time a person may receive the medical treatment he needs.

Perhaps medical care never will be a right in this country, not in the truest and fullest sense of the word. For we are never going to have enough money or manpower to place a major medical center in every neighborhood, town, and village. The family living in a remote area of rural America will always be at a relative disadvantage compared with the person living in the large urban centers. But certainly the least we can do is to make it possible for everyone in this country to seek out and receive medical care with the same sense of entitlement, so that the migrant worker can go to a doctor or enter the hospital with the same sense of security and dignity as a United States senator, and so nobody in this country ever has to worry again about collection agencies, hospital attorneys, or bankruptcy courts.

A national health insurance program of this kind might not alter the actual practice of medicine in any dramatic, sudden, or sweeping way. We could pass this program tomorrow and have no assurances that we will see radically different patterns of organization and delivery or that there will be any major change in the provider-patient relationship. These can only occur over time. Yet it is absolutely essential for us to understand that in order for these changes to even *begin* to occur, we must first change our entire frame of reference with regard to the financing of medical care. And that requires a policy decision first, and a program second. The policy decision must be a commitment to make the health of the American people public business, a commitment that nobody in this country is going to go without medical care or fear medical care because he lacks the money. When seen in this context, the two major objections to such a program, though serious, are not insurmountable.

148

The first is that it is simply too expensive, that it will cost anywhere from $70 to $100 billion a year, and that, in the current economic and political climate, the Congress just isn't going to adopt that kind of program. That may be true. But whether the Congress adopts it or not, the people of this country are still going to be spending the money. So the price tag is a false issue. The real issue is whether we want to count these billions of dollars as public expenditures, whether we think the people of this country can best be served and protected by purchasing their health insurance through the private market, with its fragmented coverage, its limited regulation, and its lack of accountability, or whether we think that a federally funded program (though not necessarily federally administered, as Senator Kennedy proposes) is the best hope of achieving the equality that we seek.

The second objection is that it is too much too soon, that we need to make improvements in other areas before taking such a major step in health insurance. We need to turn out more doctors and more paramedical personnel and drastically overhaul our current system of organization and delivery. Desirable though that may be, it might just be the one way to ensure that we will *never* have national health insurance. It is the traditional argument of the providers of care: let's have only that amount of change we are willing to tolerate, and we'll tell you when we're ready. That is not good enough. The providers can always accept more than they say they can. We are going to have to gamble on this issue. And the gamble is that once the federal government commits itself to paying the bills, it can no longer afford to be as casual about costs as it once was, as vague about the development of medical manpower, as haphazard about new forms of organization and delivery.

I am not arguing for perfection. I fully expect that once we have a program of universal entitlement, we still will be faced with problems of cost, distribution, and delivery. But assume this country did nothing more than pay the bills and institute some cost controls and professional accountability. Assume that we financed this system through general revenues, with each taxpayer paying according to his ability to pay and not according to the amount of care he received or needed. Assume that the man who is making $10,000 a year no longer pays the same monthly amount for health insurance as the executive making $60,000. Assume that heads of families in this country no longer have to face the fact that if they lose their jobs during tight economic conditions they will also lose their medical benefits. Would we call that a failure, or not enough? We might say either, but we shouldn't.

Every country that has moved to a program of national health insurance has done so pretty much within the context of its traditional political system.

Sweden, with an extensive history of local autonomy dating back to ancient times, has some twenty-five provincial or county councils that are legally responsible for providing hospital care for its citizens. More than that, health care is one of the principal purposes of local government. Much of the Swedish hospital system came about as a result of the initiative of these local authorities. There is a National Board of Health and Welfare, responsible for nationwide planning with regard to the scope, direction, and general expansion of health care services, including the supply of doctors and other trained personnel. But the actual business of program administration is done at the local or county level.

Canada, the country that is closest to the United States in area, diversity, and government structure, went the same route. The federal government passed the basic legislation, but the actual plans, and even the decision about whether to participate, was left to the discretion of the ten Canadian provinces.

While it would be a mistake for the United States to permit the fifty states to decide whether they wanted to participate in a national health insurance program, or the extent to which they wanted to participate, there is an important lesson here. It is that many national health insurance programs are not as centralized as we think, that it is entirely possible, and perhaps even desirable, to have centralized financing with decentralized administration.

Personally, I have always doubted the wisdom of a national health insurance program dominated as thoroughly by the federal government as the current system is dominated by the decisions of the private marketplace. I have doubted that such a program would have the flexibility to adapt to regional and local differences, that it would be responsive to the complaints and problems of individual patients.

Instead of turning the whole program over to the federal government or the private insurance industry, a wiser course would seem to be to let each state make its own decision on how the programs ought to be administered. The governor and the legislature could select whatever agency they wished to do the job. They could choose a Blue Cross carrier, a commercial company, a combination, or an existing state agency, or they could establish a semi-independent public corporation. The choice would be theirs. But the program would have to meet federal standards of entitlement, administration, cost control, and quality control.

At a minimum, federal standards should include uniform budgeting and reporting systems so that the performance of the states, the administrative agencies, and individual institutions, such as hospitals, or medical foundations that contract to provide services to a specified population group, could be compared, monitored, and evaluated. In the same context, the performance of individual practitioners ought to come under much greater scrutiny. Any state would be free to change its administrative arrangement at any time. The federal government would have the power to move in and administer a state program itself if the state failed to meet its obligation and responsibility. That should occur only as a last resort.

A joint federal-state health insurance plan, with the federal government collecting the money and setting the standards and with the state government administering the program and assuming the responsibility for meeting the medical care needs of all the people in its jurisdiction, is not the perfect solution, or the ideal institutional arrangement, mostly because there are no such entities as perfect institutional arrangements. No matter what system of administration the country chooses, we will still have the same employees for the most part. The expertise gained by people who worked for private insurance carriers or Blue Cross plans is not going to be squandered on the theory that we can start from scratch with another set of experts. Whatever biases they have they will continue to have or, similarly, whatever freedom they lacked to adopt a more publicly oriented course they might have in a new setting.

By allowing for regional variation and experiment, by allowing for continual review and at least the possibility of somebody else taking over the system, by allowing the health care issue to be politicized to the point where a governor would have to run for reelection on his administration of the program, concern for satisfying the consumer would be heightened.

Yet heightened interest for the consumer is nowhere near enough. The consumer doesn't need "interest." He needs a place to go, a complaint bureau, an ombudsman who works for him instead of for the providers, an office and a staff that takes him seriously and investigates his complaints. For this reason, a federal "inspector general" for medical care must be an essential part of any program that is passed.

Representatives of his office would be located in most communities. Their sole purpose would be to receive and focus on the concerns and complaints of patients. Problems would be reported directly to the governor or those charged with administering the program. Under no circumstances should the "inspector general" be an employee of the state. His independence is critical, and his judgment an important factor in helping the federal authorities assess the performance of each program.

In the long run, the office of "inspector general" might well be the most important change we bring to the American medical care system. For years, all of us in the Congress have received mail every day from people who are dissatisfied or angry with some aspect of the medical care they have received. They do not write us because they have any strong sense that we can correct what happened to them in the past. They write us because in the American medical care system there simply is no place else for them to turn. They have been rebuffed by the hospital, the insurance carrier, the doctor, and the medical society. More than anything else, the American patient needs to feel that his voice counts, that he can speak up, that he can influence the medical care system.

That is the basic outline: federal financing of universal entitlement; state administration according to federal standards; a federal "inspector general" responsible to the patients. It offers major change while allowing us flexibility and variety. It includes checks and balances on the providers of medical care and gives the patient a place where he can express his satisfaction or dissatisfaction.

It is a program that, if passed this year, could not be

implemented for another two or three years. We will need every bit of that time to think through the details of administering the program and to run some pilot projects. For there is much that we need to define, discuss, and negotiate, let alone resolve.

For example, there is the question of how much money the country wants to spend on medical care and how the money should be budgeted. An implicit assumption of any federally financed national health insurance program is that the sky is no longer the limit for the cost of medical care. A ceiling will be set, because a ceiling must be set. The country simply cannot afford to take the unquestioned word of the providers of care about the amount of money they need to provide the care and the facilities each institution says it must have.

Deciding how to set the ceiling wouldn't be too difficult. It could be set in a variety of ways: a fixed percentage of the gross national product, adjusted as the cost of living goes up or down; by an annual vote of the Congress in much the same manner that all other public funds are appropriated; in the form of an Internal Revenue Service trust fund, like the Social Security trust fund, in which a fixed percentage will be set aside for personal medical services.

Deciding how much to spend, however, will be an enormously complex and painstaking process. It will require each state to conduct an inventory of its medical care needs and resources: the cost of meeting those needs in terms of how medical care is currently organized and delivered, and the cost of meeting those needs if medical care were organized and delivered in a different manner.

Hospitals, for example, could no longer be viewed as untouchable institutions, having no particular relationship to the community as a whole. They would have to become part of an overall pattern of medical care. Eventually, this could mean that special services would be centralized in a few institutions, and smaller hospitals, perhaps around 250 to 300 beds, would become the major resource of the community. For there is some evidence that once a hospital gets beyond this size, its costs go up astronomically.

Physicians, in particular, would have to decide how they are going to bring medical services to those people who do not have them, or do not have what they need. That is no easy matter, either. But the decision will have to be made. For nobody can be permitted to go without medical care for whatever reason. That is a responsibility doctors are going to have to accept.

On the basis of this statewide inventory, negotiations would then begin between the federal government and the states about how the individual state's budget for personal health services would be calculated: what expenses would be reimbursed, which would not; whether money would be allocated strictly on a per capita basis, with a price on the head of each citizen, or whether a formula should be worked out in which money is distributed by the type of medical service in an effort to develop a more efficient system of care.

Much of this can be done only through trial and error.

But we can learn from some demonstration projects. Before the program becomes fully operational, we ought to run pilot programs in several states, have a shakedown cruise, try out various methods of reimbursement, administration, and cost control as they apply to hospitals and individual physicians. What happens, for example, when coinsurance and deductibles are a part of the program? Does this increase or decrease the use of medical services, or does it make no difference at all? Would there be any major difference between state plans administered by Blue Cross, a commercial carrier, or a public corporation? What kinds of cost controls are likely to be effective in the long run, and which look good on paper but have no practical applicability?

Another question that could be answered by trying out the program in a few states is what kinds of problems patients encounter, or feel most helpless to deal with, once the cost of care is no longer a principal worry. The answer to this and any of the above questions would be a basic resource in devising the federal standards and guidelines for both the states and the providers of care.

In conducting such experiments, we could easily find that the most "efficient" medical care would not necessarily be the best. So much of our national concern about medical care has centered on the cost of care that we often think that money is the only issue. It's not. Basically, we are trying to define the kinds of medical services that ought to be available to any individual and the manner in which they ought to be made available. However we analyze medical care, it still comes down to a decision about what is supposed to happen when a person is ill and in need of professional services. That being the case, and since we will inevitably make mistakes whatever we do, let us at least have the wisdom to err on the side of generosity.

Just as finding a problem is not the same as devising a program, so devising a program is not the same as passing a program. And unfortunately, there is a predictable pattern that social issues follow in America. We in Congress pick a problem, talk it up, offer some solutions, and then, just as we are on the verge of major legislative action, find an excuse to settle for much less than we said we needed. That is what has come to be known as a credibility gap, promising more than we had any intention of delivering, and why more and more Americans are disenchanted with their government.

That is also just about where this country happens to be with regard to national health insurance. When the issue was an abstraction several years ago, there was widespread agreement that it was an idea whose time was coming. At last the United States would catch up with the rest of the world and begin to protect its citizens against the high cost of medical care. More than that, we had at last discovered the one issue that affected *both* the poor and the middle class. Here was that elusive "unity" issue, the one where we politicians could at last do something for everybody, solving the problems of 208 million people in one fell swoop.

It was irresistible. Bills were drafted right and left. Everybody was off and running. The great American health sweepstakes were under way. Yet as national health insurance has moved from an idea whose time was coming to an idea whose time has come, the more cautious and fearful we have become. We seem to be waiting for a sign that the problems are not as serious as we once said.

Perhaps this country will not have a national health insurance program for many years to come. For we have been limping along with less than we needed in every other area of our national life, such as housing, employment, education, crime and justice, even food programs. Why should medical care strike a chord in our national conscience that other issues have not?

In a very real sense, the country that can accept hungry children as a part of its life may easily accept as a part of its life the lack of medical care, or people pushed to financial and emotional disaster because of medical bills. Will a Congress that has responded to the increasing cost of the Medicare program by making the elderly pay a larger portion of their medical bills instead of by putting the squeeze on the providers suddenly reverse its course and exact a greater standard of professional and financial accountability from doctors, hospitals, and nursing homes? At some point, we have to stop blaming the doctors, the hospitals, the insurance carriers for all the ills of American medicine. At some point, we have to start looking at Washington, to the fact that those of us in Congress are in the same position as Pogo, the comic-strip philosopher, when he said, "We have met the enemy, and he is us."

Ever since the country rediscovered the doctor shortage, the medical profession has vigorously argued that doctors shouldn't be forced to practice in areas where they didn't want to live, or be compelled to specialize in fields that held no particular interest for them. The best we could do, many physicians told me, was provide more money for medical schools to increase their enrollments, offer incentives for physicians to practice in doctor-short areas upon graduation, and hope that the trend toward "family medicine" took root so that American families would have more comprehensive medical care in the future than they have had in the past. That might not solve everybody's problem, but it clearly was an improvement upon the present situation. And if it wasn't a perfect solution, at least it was a realistic one.

Essentially, that is the place the country arrived at late in 1971. The health manpower bills the Ninety-second Congress developed and passed, and the President signed, established an open and direct relationship between federal aid to medical education and increased student enrollment in the hope that there would be about 100,000 more doctors in practice by the end of the decade than there are at the present time. The process is relatively simple. Schools of medicine, osteopathy, and dentistry that increase their student enrollments a certain percentage will receive a cash bonus for each student. During the first three years, a student would be worth $2,500 a year to the school. No payment is made for the fourth year of schooling. Upon graduation, though, the student's school receives an extra $4,000. If the student graduates at the end of three years, the school receives $6,000. Overall, it means that students who graduate in three years are worth $13,500 to their schools, and those who graduate after four years are worth $11,500. An extra bonus would go to schools that boosted enrollment beyond the mandatory amount.

In other key provisions, the legislation established (1) a new scholarship program of up to $5,000 a year for low-income students, or students living in areas without doctors who agreed to practice primary care in those areas for a period of time after graduation; (2) a new program of grants to hospitals for residency programs in family medicine; and (3) a broad program of special project grants for medical school innovations ranging from curriculum reform to creating a better distribution of medical manpower.

The bill was not without its critics. Medical schools generally felt that putting a price on each student's head would cause them severe administrative problems, and some fairly strong concern was voiced that paying the schools to increase their enrollment was money down the drain since most schools, despite their well-publicized financial troubles, could increase their output of doctors without any additional money.

Telescoping medical education into three years drew its share of fire on the grounds that it would produce more doctors only during the first year, and, furthermore, with medical knowledge increasing so rapidly, the place to cut back wasn't during the four years of medical school but during the four years of premedical school. Another reservation about the bill dealt with its heavy emphasis on physicians at the apparent expense of the allied health professions, where the need for assistance was just as acute. Also, the basic question of whether the legislation would put all medical schools on a more solid and more equitable financial foundation was left up in the air. Extra federal support might result in cutbacks of other kinds of support, such as that provided by state government.

Yet whether or not one shared the view of the critics, the legislation as a whole represented a fairly basic change in national policy. Having supported medical education through the back door in the forms of research grants to individual departments and medical school faculty members since World War II, the Congress had at last chosen to support medical education for its own sake, largely in response to the growing frustration of individuals in finding a regular doctor. With a delivery system that was lagging behind that of other countries, the time clearly seemed to have arrived for the country to put its money behind the most basic of all medical needs—producing the practicing physician.

How this is all going to work out is something we aren't really going to know much about until 1980. In the meantime, there are going to be lots of different hurdles to clear, not the least of which is financial. Money may not be the answer to all of our problems, but it's better than whatever is in second place. And the history of federal funding of medical education, like the history of federal funding of any kind of social legislation, is not one of the Congress's strong suits. We can argue that we don't get much leadership from the executive branch on occasion—President Nixon's original request was for only about 65 percent of the money authorized by the 1971 legislation—but that really isn't much of an excuse. The real truth is that we just haven't regarded medical manpower as a very important issue.

In fact, Dr. James A. Shannon, the former director of the National Institutes of Health, made that point very forcefully in comments he prepared for my Senate subcommittee's 1970 study, *The Federal Role in Health.* After reviewing the responses of the twenty-four separate departments and agencies that spent the federal health dollar—twelve of which were engaged in health training and education—Dr. Shannon drew the following conclusion:

> There seems to be no high-level appreciation of the fact that the shortage is truly great and is likely to become much greater in the immediate future. More importantly, there appears to be a lack of general awareness that the simple and modest extension of the present programs, even when coupled with new programs aimed at the evolution of new carrers (i.e., physician assistants), will not resolve the combination of short-

age and maldistribution in any reasonable period
of time.

Increasing the number of doctors and nurses graduated each year could help, Dr. Shannon pointed out, "but
only if there were specific control of their deployment."

That, of course, was the issue the 1971 manpower
legislation, for all its advances, didn't really come to
grips with.

With a little bit of luck, the legislation's incentives for
improving the distribution of doctors, both by geography and according to medical specialty, might have some
effect, particularly if the new breed of medical student
lives up to his advance billing once he gets into practice.
The trend toward group practice and health maintenance organizations should also ease the pressure,
though both their appeal and their effect may not be as
overwhelming as some of their staunchest advocates
regularly insist. But on the whole, handling the distribution problem is beyond our capacity at this particular
moment.

Which brings us right back to the issue of "forcing"
the doctor; or, putting it another way, of whether the
organization and delivery of medical care, which is what
the distribution problem really comes down to, can be
solved on as voluntary a basis as physicians would like.
The answer is no. In saying this, I am not contemplating,
proposing, or endorsing a national health service. I am
saying that if we are to fulfill our national responsibility
to bring an acceptable level of medical services within

reach of all our citizens, there are two additional measures we ought to consider.

The first is a two-year period of compulsory national service for all persons graduating from medical school or from other health care institutions; or for doctors finishing residency programs. This would be in lieu of military service. There are millions of Americans, not all of them poor, who are living in conditions that every doctor I know would call a medical emergency. Some have no doctors. Some have no surgeons. Some have unqualified people administering anesthesia. All need help. Until such time as this nation begins to organize its medical manpower and resources on a more rational and equitable basis, an emergency service seems entirely appropriate and totally necessary. Past efforts along this line have emphasized a voluntary program or the use of Public Health Service doctors and civil servants. Though these have helped, the number of requests for medical manpower has been twice as great as the number of applicants who want to serve in the program.

Moreover, it is basically unfair to place the burden for providing health and medical services on the backs of those students who cannot afford to pay for their medical education. Programs that offer scholarships to students from doctor-short areas and low-income families if they return to their neighborhoods and towns and practice medicine for a period of time—and ask nothing of students who don't need scholarships or don't live in those areas—do just that. Providing medical services is a national responsibility, one in which all young professionals ought to participate. I don't make this suggestion lightly. Similar programs ought to exist in other situations where people need the special skills that only the professional can provide.

Secondly, the federal government should begin a series of studies and negotiations with the various specialty boards, from family practice right on up to neurosurgery, to try and determine what the future of medical manpower ought to look like. One reason the United States is so top-heavy on surgeons and so lacking in anesthesiologists is that we rarely attempt to influence the professional direction of young doctors. Everybody is on his own when it comes to specialization. If the number of residency programs and positions were limited to certain specialties and locations, with the numbers, the specialties, and the locations being revised every five years, we might be able to start solving the problem of distribution both by specialty and by geography. I do not underestimate the complexity of that task. Yet we can no longer avoid the fundamental issue involved—the responsibility of the medical profession to serve the nation.

The medical corpsman has always occupied an ambiguous role in our health care system. While we were willing to trust our servicemen who were wounded in battle to carefully trained people who were not doctors, we always seemed to balk at developing the civilian equivalent of the medical corpsman. But when corpsmen began returning from Vietnam at the same time the country became aware of its doctor shortage, the whole idea was seen in a new light. Suddenly we began to realize this was a medical resource we had virtually ignored. Moreover, there wasn't any reason why a medical career of this kind shouldn't be open to people without their having first to enter the armed services.

There are about eighty programs in various stages of development that involve physicians' assistants and another fifty that seek to expand and redefine the role of the nurse. While it is too soon to make any flat prediction about how these programs will affect the doctor shortage and medical manpower generally, it is clear that there are many medical care functions that can be performed by people who are not M.D.s. These can range all the way from taking a medical history to possessing special skills in a particular area, such as baby care, or to performing a broad range of activities under the personal supervision of a doctor. Many problems still need to be resolved, such as licensing, legal liability, and public acceptance. But the physician's assistant provides a new type of medical manpower and a new avenue of access to health care delivery that could result in fundamental improvements in our medical care system.

Getting It All Together

IN THE COURSE of preparing this book, I conducted an informal survey among doctors, hospital officials, and health care planners I met. I asked them if they knew of a single community in the United States that could serve as a model of what health and medical care ought to be like, of what, in the midst of all the criticism and ferment, we were seeking as an end, or even an interim, result.

For there were many theoretical models of how health and medical services ought to be organized, and I was curious if, as health care had heated up as a public issue during the past several years, enough heat had been generated to push some of the theory off the drawing boards and out onto the streets. The answer was no. There wasn't a community of any appreciable size, such as a metropolitan area, that had taken all the different people, institutions, agencies, and functions involved in medical care and put them together into a delivery system that others would do well to emulate. There wasn't even a community that had made a good start. Occasionally, you could find a small town with only one hospital that had been able to come close, but examples like that had about as much relationship to the crucial problems of American medicine as the highly touted but extremely isolated "new towns" had to solving the problems faced by our major cities. I drew a blank. Nobody had gone much beyond the blueprint stages.

Though that was pretty much what I had expected to find, because we really hadn't paid much attention to health care organization and delivery in this country and weren't even too sure how we would reorganize medical care if we had the chance, I still was disappointed. I knew, better than most, how slow, complex, and difficult the process of major social change really was, how tedious and frustrating trying to change attitudes and behavior patterns built up over generations could become. But I also knew that we simply were not going to make much headway in developing medical care systems of the future if all we could do was *think* in community-wide terms. Somebody, somewhere, had to take some action, had to begin assessing the health and medical needs of his community, develop a set of priorities, and then begin to respond to those priorities in a concrete manner.

In particular, a way had to be found of finessing, or cracking, the autonomy and independence many actors on the medical care scene wore more as a badge of virtue than of service. Because while medicine might not resemble a cottage industry anymore in physical appearance—not with all the modern hospitals, computer technology, organ transplants, and large medical office buildings—politically speaking, it was every bit the cottage industry it had been since the first doctor treated the first patient in the colony of Virginia in 1608. That crucial element had remained unchanged. Although almost four hundred years had passed, there still was no way to come to grips with American medicine as a profession or health care as an industry, nothing anyone could get a handle on. Each unit, institution, and person went its or his own way, all answering only to themselves and insisting that they were the only ones capable of deciding when, if, and how they should change.

Medicine had put the lie to the poet. Every doctor *was* an island. And so was every hospital. Which meant that even if some board, agency, or group of private citizens came up with a rough approximation of how a community's medical resources might be used more effectively and fairly, they had a better chance of flying to the moon than making their decision stick. Thus, the trappings of change and community-wide efforts were often present. But since nobody had or was particularly willing to exert any political muscle over anybody else, everything rested on moral authority, persuasion, and appeals to better instincts. It wasn't enough.

The experience of one large Eastern city with which I am familiar illustrates the point.

Largely through the initiative of a few hospital trustees, an organization was formed in this city in mid-1970 for the purpose of establishing and coordinating a community-wide network of prepaid group practice plans. Anywhere from ten to twenty medical groups were anticipated, with all of them using existing facilities to cut down the costs of the program, and with the program being marketed through existing insurance carriers. If successful, the network would make that city the only one in America to offer all its residents a choice on how they wanted to receive their medical care. They could continue the predominant method of purchasing insurance for hospital care and then paying their private doctors on a fee-for-service basis. Or they could choose to enroll in a prepaid group practice and pay a fixed sum every month that would cover all their basic doctor and hospital bills.

All the major hospitals, medical societies, physician groups, insurance carriers, and medical schools were invited to participate. So were the representatives of business and labor, consumer groups, and social agencies. The theory was that if the new organization could establish this kind of broad-based support at the start—each participant had to pay an initiation fee as a demonstration of his commitment—there was a better than even chance the idea would work and the network could be put together. The response was heartening. Nearly sixty different organizations paid their money to take their chances.

Fully aware of the pitfalls that lay in store, the organizers carefully planned their next steps and gave themselves a generous target date. They were in no hurry, preferring something that would work over the long haul than something that could show instant results and then fizzle away. If, by the end of two years, they had some medical groups organized and were treating patients, they would be satisfied.

That would also signal the time to disband the original organization and replace it with a wholly new consumer-oriented corporation that would function as the permanent community-wide umbrella agency. "Consumer-oriented" meant a majority of the board would come from the general public and not from medicine or medical institutions. The new corporation would not provide any medical services directly. Its duties would be limited to contracting with the medical groups, establishing standards, guidelines, and criteria of performance, coordinating the network, and monitoring the operation of the whole program.

Once it was under way, though, the problems started filtering in. Business and industry weren't giving the support many felt they should. The suburban doctors didn't want any part of prepaid group practice. There was a basic conflict between doctors and hospitals, because any program that gave doctors incentives to use less expensive services went directly against the hospitals, who were used to having their beds filled and their laboratories and special facilities going full blast.

And so, after a year, there wasn't a patient in sight because there wasn't a medical group in sight except for the one that had existed in an outlying town before the program began and a neighborhood health center that also preceded the program. Plans were rescaled and target dates reset. Perhaps a smaller start could be made, such as having some hospital-based group practices in areas where large numbers of poor and elderly lived without regular medical services and used the hospital emergency room as a family doctor.

The motivation wasn't quite as pure as it sounded. The emergency rooms and outpatient departments were losing money. By working out an arrangement with state and federal officials to cover Medicaid and Medicare patients on a prepaid basis, the hospitals hoped to do better than they had under the fee schedule of both programs. Never mind, though. At least it was an incentive for changing and for doing what many felt was the right thing.

No luck. And at sixteen months, the organizers were hoping they might have something going in another two years. "We misread the situation," explained one of the participants. "It turned out to be a Council of Kings. Staying away would have been bad public relations, so everybody came and said all the right things. But they were coming mostly to protect their own turf, to make sure nobody imposed anything upon them they didn't want. And in medicine, or anything else, when your main interest is preventing encroachment, you don't get very far. Defense may be the name of the game in football, but in a human service, it can destroy you."

Events at one of the hospitals involved, and the only one at this writing likely to produce doctors for a new medical group, offered an additional behind-the-scenes look at medical politics in just one institution, let alone throughout a whole community.

Essentially, they had the same experience as the community-wide organization. Two senior members of the medical staff, a surgeon and a urologist, convinced that a hospital-based prepaid group practice was the only way to provide personal and continuing medical care for the 25,000 residents of the surrounding neighborhoods, took their case to the board of trustees. They argued that the emergency room and outpatient departments were hardly satisfactory replacements for the doctors who had left the area, and that the need was further proven by the fact that, on any given day, at least 35 percent of the patients who had been admitted to the hospital had no regular physician of their own. The doctors asked for $30,000 to renovate the outpatient department, to rip out the benches and turn the facility into a comfortable and attractive suite of waiting rooms, examining rooms, and doctors' offices. The board voted the money.

The entire medical staff was the next stop. To their surprise, the two doctors found that every member of the seventy-man medical staff wanted to be a charter member and would donate $100 to the organization.

That unanimity was short-lived. When committees were appointed to work out a particular problem, nobody showed up. When the organizers said they wanted to eliminate all the various clinics that had sprung up over the years and bring everything "under one roof," doctors who had a personal and financial stake in maintaining their clinics as independent entities wanted out. When the medical staff learned each person would have to donate at least three continuous hours of time a week, 90 percent said that was all the time they had to give to the project. When they learned that all money collected would go to the group, there was more internal dissension.

Within a few months, the project was abandoned. Everything had fallen apart before anything could get off the ground. "Democracy was our downfall," one of the original physicians said in retrospect. "We let any active member join and got about ten guys who were committed and sixty who were hedging a bit, who were willing to lose $100 to have some veto power. Our idea was to treat people as they would be treated in a private office, to eliminate individual clinics. And the minute we did that, the docs said we were accusing them of practicing bad medicine. We weren't. We were accusing them of practicing behind the times, of not realizing that everybody is entitled to personal medical care. Physicians have thought that the way to take care of a poor person is to treat him in a poor clinic in a poor way. They didn't want their patients bothering them. They wanted patients who would get sick at a certain time on a certain day—during clinic. They didn't want patients telephoning them or seeking help the other six days and twenty-one hours of the week.

"The patients didn't even realize they could do this. They had no sense of what their rights were, of how to go about getting medical care. We wanted to instill in them a generous chunk of expectation, let them learn what it was like to be a private patient."

There's a silver lining of sorts. The two doctors regrouped, found another five who were sympathetic, and, with the $30,000 still available for remodeling, put together a group that will offer some comprehensive care for the neighborhood. It won't be prepaid. They're not big enough. But they hope that by starting out on a fee-for-service basis, they can grow into a prepaid group, especially when Medicaid and Medicare begin covering subscribers on a capitation (per person) basis. Besides the surgeon and the urologist, the group will have two family practitioners, an orthopedist, a pediatrician, and an obstetrician-gynecologist.

They also hope to bring the two general practitioners left in the neighborhood into the program by offering them backup services at the hospital and making a family health worker available to them in the office. If that arrangement works out, the family health worker will begin to make house calls, encouraging residents to come in for preventive medicine and checkups, and following up those who have already received treatment.

Measured against what the community-wide organization hoped to accomplish—and the proposal shouldn't be written off this soon—the results are extremely meager. They do not offer much hope of changing the patterns of medical care in the near future. The plans and visions are fine, but they seem to be on a level we cannot come close to matching with our real-world efforts. And in the end, we wind up doing what we had desperately hoped to avoid: settling for what we could get, for six doctors instead of none, one group practice instead of none, one hospital instead of none; and wondering how long the scraps of social change can keep alive the spirit of social change.

And yet . . .

Is settling for what we can get so deplorable in every case? Have our efforts during the past several years been so inadequate? Have we really produced nothing more than scraps? Can we afford to reject changes because they do not occur on the scale we want and at the pace we want?

Focusing so exclusively on our failures, on what we have not accomplished, can be just as unrealistic as being mesmerized by success stories. A great deal of change has occurred in American medicine recently, more than most of us realize. Only it's not apparent when we look for the one community that has solved *all* its problems, or achieved a level of problem-solving unmatched by anyone else.

If, however, we lower our sights somewhat and forego the cosmic view for some programs and alternatives that have worked in different places, the future doesn't look nearly as bleak. There are successful prepaid group practices. There are medical care foundations, which are groups that preserve fee-for-service payment. There are neighborhood health centers in the ghetto, rural health care projects, hospitals that have begun to share facilities and services, computer technology that offers a more efficient and accurate brand of medicine, and the growing trend toward using physicians' assistants and paramedical personnel.

Perhaps none of these has, by itself, produced any major, basic, or fundamental change in American medicine. But they have improved the ability of physicians to provide medical care. They have made medical care available in places where none existed before. They have resulted in medical institutions assuming a greater social responsibility than they had in the past. And they have resulted in physicians beginning to question traditional methods of practice, organize themselves in groups, and work as part of a medical team that includes non-physicians as well.

Some examples:

• In Decorah, Iowa, four specialists—a surgeon, a radiologist, a pathologist, and a psychiatrist—travel to seven other towns on a regular basis, providing services for small hospitals that cannot attract full-time staff people.

• Some residents of Rochester, New York, are about to have a choice of two more kinds of medical care instead of being limited to the customary solo fee-for-service brand that always existed. The medical society is establishing a medical care foundation, while Blue Cross and the hospitals have joined together to sponsor a prepaid group practice.

• In Flemington, New Jersey, the Hunterdon Medical Center, which was one of the first hospitals in the country to establish family practice residencies, has put two family practitioners on its payroll so they can provide medical care in a small doctorless town in one of the poorest sections of the county. Plans are under way for the hospital to sponsor doctors in two other towns as well.

• In the Columbia Point section of Boston, the Watts section of Los Angeles, and the south Bronx section of New York City, neighborhood health centers are an integral part of the community. The Watts center alone employs some forty to fifty doctors of all specialties, and the Martin Luther King Health Center in the south Bronx has used neighborhood residents to conduct community health surveys on a door-to-door basis and act as "ombudsmen" for families who need both social and medical services.

• In Salem, Missouri, a remote village in the Ozark Mountains, Dr. Billy Jack Bass has an "automated physician's assistant." It's a teletype machine that permits him to transmit information about his own patients to the Missouri Regional Medical Program office 130 miles away. The RMP has an IBM computer that can store 10 million pages of medical information, and other useful technological items, that is linked directly to Dr. Bass's office. Patients can now receive a complete physical without leaving town. They once traveled a hundred miles and spent three days to get one.

• Phoenix, Arizona, has a couple of new developments going for it. One is the Surgicenter, a building that houses four operating rooms and one recovery room and where minor operations can be performed on an outpatient basis. It's an alternative to high-cost hospitalization in cases where the medical need does not warrant that kind of expense. The other is the establishment of an eight-hospital corporation for the purpose of improving the efficiency and management of all eight. Represented by a single board, the Samaritan Health Service began its operations by sharing personnel and entering into joint purchase agreements.

The number of people and institutions involved in these and similar changes, or receiving their benefits, is probably fairly small. But it's worth noting that much of what we consider worthwhile in medicine today had the same kind of start and took many years to develop. Under national health insurance, more political clout will exist so that what seems impossible to achieve on a broader scale today may be easier to achieve tomorrow. Meanwhile, if we are seriously interested in changing American medicine, or in learning what experiences we can draw upon, there are many other examples that also merit close attention. Two that have made a special impression on me are a University of Florida program in rural health care delivery, and the Group Health Cooperative of Puget Sound in Seattle, Washington.

Of all the medical care problems in this country, none is more serious, or more shameful, than our inability to provide care for the rural poor. Regardless of what happens in the city, at least there are emergency rooms and outpatient departments people can get to without too much trouble. The rural poor, on the other hand, are often totally isolated. There is no place for them to go and nobody who is coming to them.

So when Dr. Harry Prystowsky was invited to leave his teaching-research post at The Johns Hopkins University College of Medicine in Baltimore, Maryland, to become chairman of the Department of Obstetrics and Gynecology at the University of Florida College of Medicine in Gainesville, Florida, he began asking himself a series of questions. What, Dr. Prystowsky wondered, *is* the role of a single academic department in providing community health and medical services? Is it useful for an academic department to participate in "extramural" health programs? Can the department have any important impact if it undertakes such efforts?

That was in 1958, and the answers were a long time coming. But by the end of 1971, Dr. Prystowsky had them in the form of a health and medical services program his department had developed for the rural poor, specifically for women and children. Moreover, the program had grown to the point where it was delivering health and medical care in thirteen counties and across 10,000 square miles, an area roughly the size of the state of Maryland; and the state of Florida had sounded out the department about putting together a statewide program.

As for numbers, which have been the customary way of measuring success, during the past four years alone some 90,000 patients received treatment in the program's twenty-three clinics. Another 12,000 received hospital care at the W. A. Shands Hospital, the teaching hospital of the University of Florida. They included 4,600 women who were pregnant and had given birth,

2,800 women who needed hospitalization for reasons other than pregnancies, and 4,800 newborns who needed special services and treatment.

In point of fact, the program is a cooperative effort between the University of Florida, the county health departments, and the Florida Division of Health. And ironically, the idea of providing services over a thirteen-county area came not from Dr. Prystowsky or anyone else in the medical school. It came from the state. In 1965, when the federal government first began funding maternal and infant care programs, the state of Florida, aware of Dr. Prystowsky's success over a three-county area, asked him how he felt about entering into a contract with them to develop a maternity program for the thirteen counties of north-central Florida. Dr. Prystowsky didn't hesitate for a moment. Here, if the university was willing, was the chance he had waited for, the opportunity to develop a health maintenance program for women and begin delivering comprehensive health and medical care to at least one group among the rural poor. The university was willing. So were the county health departments.

Though the county health departments furnish the clinic space, usually their own offices, the basic component of the program is the mobile health manpower teams organized, trained, and dispatched by Dr. Prystowsky's department. Each team is headed by a resident physician and also includes a county public health nurse, a social worker, a nutritionist, a community "outreach" worker, a medical student, and sometimes a clerk. Among them, they are able to provide a basic level of health, medical, and social services or arrange for those they cannot provide themselves.

A major objective of the program is to bring the services to the people. That means a heavy responsibility falls upon the outreach workers. They are the ones who go down the dirt roads and through the backwoods, to places the public health nurses never knew about or never found, searching for women and children who need care and driving them to and from the clinic if necessary. One outreach worker recently found a baby with worms coming out of his nose. Another found an infant who had double pneumonia and who would have died within twenty-four hours if the outreach worker had not showed up at the door and rushed him to the university hospital.

Outreach workers begin their visits by engaging the women in some general conversation. How many children do they have? If there are five school-age children but two are at home, why is that? Are there only enough clothes and shoes for three children? Does the family get enough to eat? Do they need help getting clothes, food, or fuel? Have the children who are not in school received shots? And what about those who are? Did they get their shots?

Very often, a lot of conversation has to take place between an outreach worker and a woman who has never received medical care or social services, or who has no understanding of how family planning could ease the strain of her life, before the woman decides to come to the clinic. But the outreach workers are women who are in the program themselves. They are not much different from those they are visiting. They have experienced the same kinds of hardships, or at least known about them more directly and vividly than anyone else on the health care team. And they can convey a sense of concern, comfort, and friendship that often makes the difference between whether or not a woman and her children begin receiving health and medical care.

But once they do, they enter a medical care system. Each woman has a medical record and a medical history, perhaps for the first time in her life. One copy stays at the clinic closest to her home. The other is at the medical school, where cases are reviewed and studied on a regular basis. Women no longer just show up at a hospital to give birth and then go home after delivery. They come to the clinics for prenatal examinations, are guided through their pregnancies, and then give birth at the university hospital, which is located in the exact center of the thirteen-county area. A member of the health care team follows the progress of mother and child in the hospital and makes sure they continue receiving care after both are back home.

The clinics themselves are sometimes a makeshift sort of arrangement, with large rooms being curtained off into smaller ones. But great pains are taken to see that the actual care itself is both personal and private, what each member of the health care team would want for himself. Numbers are avoided like the plague. Everyone is called by name at all times. Though the women see a number of different people during the course of each visit, the services are well organized. Nobody leaves before their case and any future appointments and services that need to be arranged have been reviewed and discussed with a county public health nurse, the team member who is responsible for follow-up work between clinic sessions.

Whatever sense of pride and accomplishment the professionals on the health care team may have, it is still the outreach worker who has the greatest sense of what has happened and how far they have come. They know what it was like before. They know that, as one of them said, "we have people coming here who wouldn't have come to town if you sent them a golden chariot." They have seen the program respond to what the patients wanted, and that was something they thought they would never see. Now the nurses often give vaginal examinations, not because of any medical school theory about using medical manpower "efficiently" and having the doctor perform only the "most important" functions, but because the women were embarrassed and self-conscious about having men examine them. Because of this, Dr. Prystowsky's department has a training program in obstetrics for the nurses. Likewise, early plans for group discussion of family planning were vetoed by the patients. They wanted to talk about their problems individually, or at most with two other women. They got what they wanted.

One of the more recent developments is a group of family planning clinics in the Gainesville area staffed totally by public health nurses, outreach workers, and clerks. It is financed in part by an Office of Economic Opportunity grant in family planning. Two nurses are present at each session, and they divide their time between examining patients and interviewing them. Outreach workers have been trained to assist in the examinations. A physician is on call at all times. At first the clinic was open only in the morning. As word spread and demand for service grew, sessions at night—from 6:30 P.M. to 11:30 P.M.—were scheduled, as well as on weekends.

The program is not without its shortcomings, and Dr. Prystowsky knows them better than anyone. The first is that it serves *only* women and children. A second is that the maternal and infant care programs place limits on the length of time a person may receive care—six weeks after delivery for the mother, one year after birth for the child. That is hardly comprehensive care. A third is that the health care teams sometimes reach certain clinics only twice a month. Though the county health departments and local hospitals are available between sessions and the county public health nurses try to follow up on each case, there isn't the full continuity of care Dr. Prystowsky would like to see.

There is also a fourth shortcoming. Despite the support the program has received from federal, state, and county government, it still exists outside the mainstream of medical care in the thirteen-county area. No private physicians participate in the program. Nor do any of the community hospitals. Thus, when Dr. Prystowsky says he has the support and cooperation of the private doctors and the local medical establishments, what he seems to be saying is that they have no objection to the medical school and the county getting together to treat people they weren't treating in the first place for one reason or another. In fairness to the doctors and hospitals, though, the obstetricians and the hospital in one county chose to provide the services themselves on a reimbursement basis. They dropped out, citing the lack of time and the shortage of hospital beds.

Yet, overall, the program must be judged a success, one of the more remarkable "demonstration" projects that has come to my attention. It has shown that it is possible not only to plan a large-scale effort across a sizable geographic area, but to develop and implement the idea as well. Furthermore, while many demonstration programs are isolated from the political and social structure of the community, this one was not. Its growth and success are due in large measure to the involvement and cooperation of the university and the various levels of government. And it stands as a dramatic example of what can happen when a medical school decides to take an activist role in the delivery of health services to people who previously had received none, or had received them on a sporadic basis.

The last point deserves special emphasis. It's probably true that, in the long run, we cannot begin to solve the problem of rural medical care on any kind of lasting basis unless that solution occurs within the context of overall rural development, just as we probably cannot make similar strides in our central cities without a basic shift in our national priorities. Yet developments like that are a long way off; too long to wait for. Hungry men cannot exist on promises that, in time, all men shall feast as equals on delicacies prepared by the world's finest chefs. However attractive that may be as an ideal, hungry men would have full stomachs right now if somebody would just put up a cafeteria around the corner. And in a sense, that's where the action ought to be in many of our medical schools.

Our concern for producing more doctors and putting medical schools on a better financial footing consumed most of our attention and energy in the past few years. Now that the health manpower legislation the Congress developed and passed in 1971 has put us on the right track and has begun to put the weight of the federal government behind residency programs in family practice, it's time for both the country and the medical schools to focus on the delivery of medical services.

By bringing medical schools directly into the delivery of services, a number of things can happen. The most obvious is that people begin to receive medical care. Not so obvious, but potentially of greater significance with regard to basic changes in medicine, is what can happen to a medical student trained in this kind of academic setting.

I remember talking about this one time with a professor of internal medicine I had come to know fairly well and who had taught at three different medical schools— one on the East Coast, one in the Midwest, and one on the West Coast. I had asked him what, in his view, was the greatest single flaw in American medical education.

With characteristic bluntness, he replied, "We never teach our students the most important part of medicine. We never teach them what it's like to be a patient. So they go out into practice not knowing what patients really need and why they are so upset with us." Medical students, he said, rarely learned what medicine looked like from the bottom up because their professors made little effort to leave the ivory tower.

"Medicine isn't just a physical science," he told me. "It's a human and a social science as well. But we're not going to get that point across until medical schools themselves become involved in the delivery of care on a day-to-day basis. There's no other way. It's all back at the factory." He was right. Medical schools ought to be health care laboratories where students can become familiar with problems that exist in the communities where they are trained, and where they are going to live and practice.

There are some encouraging trends in this direction. Responding to criticism that medical students don't even see patients until their third year, the University of Missouri–Kansas City medical school, which has developed a six-year program of medical education that begins after high school, has students seeing patients on their first day. During the first two years, students spend one-quarter of their time with patients and increase that to three-quarters during the last four years. In addition, each student spends the last four years following a group of fifty patients.

In some schools, such as Georgetown University in

Washington, D.C., the Department of Community Medicine is trying to develop a prepaid group practice plan so students can learn from some direct and continuing exposure to this type of medical care.

Another change can be found at the new University of Illinois medical school in Rockford. Dr. Robert L. Evans, the dean, has brought private practitioners onto the faculty and is having faculty members provide care in towns without doctors. The purpose is to break down any town-and-gown tensions that might exist and remind the full-time faculty that what people need the most is found outside the medical school walls.

The School of Medicine of the State University of New York at Buffalo proved recently that the way to get black students into medical school was to go out and find them. In two years, the school admitted thirty-four black students, all of whom are doing well. Though the federal government now provides financial incentives for schools that increase their enrollments, Buffalo increased its enrollment without adding to its budget.

Social and institutional change is a mysterious business. We can identify the institutions and the people involved. We can select certain "leverage" points that are supposed to produce more results than others. But after that, it's pretty much a waiting game. And a long one at that. Thus, in medicine, nobody can say with any assurance whether medical schools create change or respond to it, or whether the changes that medical schools attempt to stimulate can stand up on the outside. Yet we can say that nothing, absolutely nothing, is going to change unless our medical schools change, and with them, the other institutions of medical education and service. For instinct alone tells us that medical schools exert a powerful influence on patterns of medical practice and care. It is the medical school that determines who is admitted as a medical student. It is the medical school that transmits certain basic attitudes about the profession and its responsibilities, and very often these attitudes are transmitted by osmosis more than anything else.

Osmosis? Yes, indeed. Because when Dr. Harry Prystowsky looks around the state of Florida and elsewhere (Arizona, Pennsylvania, Connecticut) these days, he sees many of his former students and residents and faculty in important positions. They are hospital chiefs of staff or department heads. They are moving up the ladder of local medical societies. And to Dr. Prystowsky's great satisfaction and delight, they are bringing the same kind of leadership to their institutions that he brought to his. The only difference is that in the current climate, change ought to occur faster than it did back in 1958.

While many health care planners spent last year cooking up visions of a medical future in which computers not only diagnosed illness but treated patients as well, the people at the Group Health Cooperative of Puget Sound in Seattle, Washington, one of the most successful prepaid group practices in the country, were wrestling with a problem that seemed almost trivial in comparison.

They were wondering whether their neighborhood medical centers, which traditionally have housed about fifteen doctors, ought to be redesigned so that only ten doctors practiced in a single location; or, failing that, so that doctors practiced only in clusters of five or ten within a single location. Though they couldn't put their finger on the exact reason, the Group Health administrative staff felt that, internally, the edges got a little ragged when a health center supporting staff had to react to fifteen different doctors. And if that was the case, they didn't want any sense of irritation or frustration filtering up and creeping into the doctor-patient relationship, particularly as they continued to grow in size and build more centers.

Technology and computers are going to shape our medical future. There's not much question about that. Yet the kind of question Group Health asked itself may turn out to be more important in the long run. For it is a reminder that no matter how much technology we develop, medicine is still a personal service. And if there is any one thought or idea that binds together all the criticism made of American medicine, it is this: medicine is too impersonal and becoming even more so.

Whether medicine has in fact become more impersonal than anything else in our society, or reflects that trend, really isn't very important. What is important is that patients feel this way and that far too many people in our society look upon medical care the way they look upon buying a car. If they get through the experience without being ambushed financially or emotionally, it's a bonus: like buying that car and finding out it's not a lemon after all.

Group Health doesn't claim its medicine is the nation's best or most personal. Like most organizations with a good story to tell, Group Health is blessed with institutional modesty. Its staff has something that works for their subscribers. They're happy to explain it to others. But they draw the line at saying they have the answer to anybody else's problems.

Regardless, Group Health is being looked to more and more as a model of what an urban health care delivery system ought to be; or what a rural one ought to be, for that matter. Its six neighborhood medical centers tied to one central hospital are fairly close to what many now believe is the inevitable trend in medicine—decentralized units of primary care feeding into a larger institution such as a hospital, and all of them contained within a single organizational unit. Currently, Group Health serves 150,000 people in the Seattle area. By the end of the decade, it will be serving 337,000 and will have a network of fourteen medical centers and three hospitals.

But that's not really why people come to look at Group Health. They come to Seattle because the Group Health Cooperative of Puget Sound is one of the few health care delivery systems in this country that is owned by consumers and controlled by consumers.

A product of the cooperative movement that flourished in the late thirties and early forties, the original capital for Group Health came from 400 families who put up $100 each in 1946. That led to the purchase one year later of a small medical clinic that was failing financially, but whose staff seemed to like the idea of prepaid medical care. For a long time, it was a fly-by-the-seat-of-the-pants operation, with organized medicine generating powerful opposition and growth occurring slowly. In the fifties, everything began to fall into place, and Group Health is now a $21-million-a-year organization that employs over 1,350 people, including 145 doctors.

Co-op membership now costs $175 a family, and more than 6,000 families have purchased an additional $8 million of 6 percent Group Health bonds to help the program expand. Growth has also brought in many members who, though selecting Group Health over other types of coverage offered at their place of employment, choose not to join the cooperative. Only about 45 percent of the subscribers are actual "owners."

Critics and competitors of Group Health concede that the plan is consumer-owned, but they say the consumer control aspect is a myth. "The same three people show up at every board meeting," and "the committees do what the doctors tell them" are two frequently voiced criticisms. Both miss the point. Consumer control and participation doesn't mean open warfare must exist between doctor and patient, that the whole organization has to be wracked with knock-down, drag-out battles that leave everybody spent and bitter. It doesn't mean that providers and consumers have to disagree on all major issues. Nor does it mean that every consumer is satisfied all of the time.

What it does mean is the existence of a mechanism and

a process whereby those who receive the care are in a position to influence that care, both on a policy-making level and as individual patients with specific problems. And at Group Health, both exist. Consumers influence policy through the eleven-member Board of Trustees, which includes one elected representative from each of the six medical centers. They make their individual voices known through a Member Relations Department that takes their complaint, brings it to the attention of the individual doctor or the appropriate Group Health Committee and tries to resolve it or make sure a repeat performance is avoided. Doctors also have a chance to complain about individual patients who, for instance, fail to keep appointments.

Now that Group Health is a quarter of a century old, there aren't any more "hot" issues like the one that threatened to split the whole program wide open early in the 1950s. A surgeon fired by the medical staff, which operates under a contract with the board, appealed to the board and was reinstated. He was eventually dropped with three months' pay. From that incident came the Joint Conference Committee, consisting of three doctors and three trustees, which resolves all potential conflicts between consumers and providers. Thus those who provide the care and those who receive the care have the opportunity to discuss their problems and work out solutions without either side feeling they have been "had" by the other. This is no small achievement.

Because Group Health is well known and attracts only doctors who want to practice in this mold, the program runs fairly smoothly to begin with. Still, the board members and consumers who participate on other committees have spent enough time at their job to have developed an expertise often lacking in board members of other institutions. At Group Health, it is not a case, as it can be elsewhere, of the doctors running the program and the board running the errands. Trustees meet every month to review all facets of program operation and to pass on recommendations made by working committees. The board hires the medical director and the hospital administrator and approves the appointment of each doctor the medical staff wants to hire. Once a year, there is a general membership meeting where co-op "owners" can vote on issues such as the cost of the plan and the kinds of items and services they would like to see included.

The membership has rejected the idea of coinsurance and deductibles on routine medical care. Their view is that medical services are there to be used, not protected, and that it is foolish, as some people suggest, to charge an extra dollar or two as a reminder not to abuse the program or the service when you go to the doctor or get a prescription filled. And they have a very comprehensive package of services. All doctor and hospital care is covered. People who need visiting nurse or home health care receive it. Drugs are included, with tranquilizers, birth control pills, and dietary supplements being the only exceptions. (Group Health is on the verge of approving a more sophisticated family planning program. But birth control pills will be available on a prepaid basis only for those low-income people whose care is government-financed. Both the cooperative members and the group subscribers voted last year not to prepay birth control pills.) Each patient is entitled to ten psychiatric visits a year, but if they make more, it costs only $5 a visit. Eye examinations are covered and glasses are provided at cost. For this, a family of four pays $44 a month.

The organization of the medical services themselves deserves comment. Long before most people were talking about the importance of primary care and of developing a new kind of specialist in family medicine, Group Health was moving in this direction. As a matter of fact, it seems to have cornered the market on general and family practitioners. They comprise a full 40 percent of the medical staff, and even the chief of staff is a general practitioner. They are the nucleus of the program and man the neighborhood medical centers, because Group Health has decided that people want and need a family doctor more than anything else. Nobody is forced to take one. People can come downtown and see a specialist if they choose. But most families like the idea of going to a single physician who knows each member of the family, can care for them both as a family and as individuals, and can guide them through the rest of the medical care system when necessary. By emphasizing this kind of relationship, Group Health hopes it can stem the tide of depersonalization that seems to be the order of the day.

Also available at each medical center are an internist, a pediatrician, an optometrist or ophthalmologist, and sometimes an obstetrician. Numbers vary with the number of people who use the center. Specialists in radiology, dermatology, pathology, anesthesiology, urology, neurology, neurosurgery, general surgery, and mental health are all downtown at the central hospital, which also contains a diagnostic center. Each medical center also has a pharmacy and an optometrist shop where glasses are made, fitted, and purchased. Physicians' assistants from the University of Washington "Medex" program, which trains returning army corpsmen for civilian medical care, are on the medical center staffs and at the emergency room at the downtown hospital. A newer development is a program within Group Health to train nurse practitioners who will also assist physicians by performing many of the more routine medical tasks.

In establishing its six neighborhood medical centers, Group Health was responding to its growth and the need of members to have medical facilities that were more convenient than the combination hospital–primary care center near the center of town. One of those centers is in a downtown office building, partly for the convenience of people working downtown but mostly because many elderly subscribers wanted doctors' offices they could reach without too much trouble. Several buses stop in front of the building that houses the downtown medical center.

All in all, a fairly complete package of medical services is available at the centers. They are open only from about 8:30 in the morning to 5:30 in the evening. After that, patients go to the combination emergency room–outpatient department at the hospital. For most subscribers, that's a twenty-minute drive at most. Driving time will be reduced when the two additional hospitals are built. Before anyone goes to the hospital, however, he calls so his medical record can be pulled out and will be ready for him. The next morning, the patient's family doctor receives a written report on the medical treatment given. Either way, patients are going to an emergency room they know and where they feel they are known even if they haven't been there before. What happens in the emergency room will become part of the patient's overall medical record, something that doesn't happen in most emergency rooms.

Group Health's liabilities are as visible as its assets. It's primarily a program for middle-class whites, even though some poor are being treated through Model City, Medicaid, and Office of Economic Opportunity grants. Complaints about "impersonal" care and long waits for appointments have become disturbingly frequent. The program has its share of dropouts (total turnover for any reason is less than 5 percent a year), as well as members who occasionally go outside the system for care even though they have to pay for it out of their own pockets.

For those who are satisfied, and they are a great majority, Group Health provides the financial and emotional security they feel their neighbors don't have. As one subscriber put it: "I never thought much about whether this is a good thing to be in. One day I saw my neighbor going into fits because he couldn't find a doctor and didn't know what to do and where to go. That was when I knew I had something good. I just don't worry about those probems anymore."

And of course there is the consumer element.

Consumer control and consumer participation are concepts and practices that are new to medicine and to the health care industry. Those who advocate them are sometimes vague about what they have in mind. There is nothing vague, however, about their feeling that one of the most unequal relationships in the country is one patient going against one medical care system. It's unequal because in most medical care systems there is no single person, no agency, no organization, no mechanism whose sole function is to represent the patient, to be his advocate, to critically evaluate the care he has received and the manner in which he has received it; in effect, to hold the system, the profession, and the industry accountable. Without this sense of representation, a patient begins to feel that the hospital or the doctor's office is just another assembly line, one more corporation and bureaucracy to deal with, one more part of his life that he must live according to the rules somebody else set for him.

Group Health is not the last word in consumerism. It's closer to the first. But it has developed a process in which the providers of care engage in an open and honest debate with the consumers of care about the kinds of authority their training qualifies them, and them alone, to exercise; and the kinds of authority it does not entitle them to exercise as completely and as privately as they have in the past. Nobody can tell a doctor how to treat a patient, and lay interference in the actual practice of medicine can have disastrous consequences. But the social and financial context in which medicine occurs and the manner in which it is organized and delivered are decisions that ought to be public decisions in the broadest possible sense.

The entire future of medicine rests on this kind of open communication between doctors and patients, or the representatives of patients. The fresh wind of secularism has blown through every other religion, and now it is blowing through medicine, which in this and most other countries, has attained a status fairly close to that of a religion. For the moment, the thrust is to place people who have no regular association with medicine or its institutions on hospital boards or on community advisory boards. There is also a growing public sentiment that there really should be no difference at all between the tax money government spends and the insurance money hospitals and doctors spend. Each is public money held in trust. Each ought to be spent according to rigid standards of public accountability and according to specific needs of the community, as determined by agencies directly responsible to the public, not agencies whose sentiments rest heavily with the hospital or the doctor.

Eventually, consumer representation ought to extend to medicine's quality control boards as well. Medicine simply cannot continue to exist in a democratic society if it maintains the fiction that in order to judge the quality of care, you must be a doctor. Yes, only doctors can treat

patients. But I cannot believe that medicine is so aston-
ishingly complex, or its standards so intricate, that a
normal, intelligent human being cannot follow the
thought processes of doctors and hospital officials. The
absence of any outside point of view is an open invitation
to intellectual rigor mortis. If I were a doctor, I would
welcome somebody who didn't know as much about
medicine as I did sitting in on my discussions, question-
ing my assumptions and my standards, and keeping my
mind open.

As for those doctors and hospitals who feel consumer
participation, representation, and involvement is unnecessary or harmful, that medicine will develop the appropriate accountability through a natural process of
evolution, I can only say that they are wrong. Consumerism is a new idea all right. But basically, it amounts to
nothing more than patients asking for what doctors and
hospitals themselves would ask for if the roles were reversed and they were on the outside looking in.

Programs such as those just described in this chapter
emphasize the talent, the imagination, and the sense of
responsibility that exist among large segments of the
medical profession. The capacity for change is present.
But how much easier it would be for everyone if government fulfilled its role and provided the basic foundations
of national health insurance and full support for the
programs that would produce the doctors and other
health care professionals this country needs.

Epilogue

SOME OF THE MOST memorable medical care I ever encountered occurred, not surprisingly, at the Mayo Clinic in Rochester, Minnesota. I had expected a medical staff superbly trained and supremely competent. I wasn't disappointed. But that wasn't what made such a lasting impression upon me. It was the manner in which the care was organized and the atmosphere in which the care was rendered. And all this happened some years before the organization and delivery of medical care came into public prominence.

My wife and I had gone to the Mayo Clinic so she could undergo a series of examinations and consultations to determine if she needed heart surgery. While she was there, I decided to get a complete physical checkup myself. It was the most impressive examination I ever had, the kind everybody in this country should have.

To begin with, though I had been instrumental in providing the Mayo Clinic with a large sum of money for an experimental hospital, I did not receive VIP treatment during the examination. I know this because the doctor in charge of the examination had just finished his residency in Canada and this was his first year at the Mayo Clinic. He was not one of the senior men on the staff. In addition, I never went to the head of the line. Like everyone else, I had a number and took my turn all the way down the line and throughout the day.

Practically the whole examination, all the tests and all the procedures, which many doctors still do by themselves, was performed by paramedical personnel and technicians. They were highly skilled and made me feel very comfortable. At the end of the day, the results were brought to the doctor in charge. He reviewed them with me, told me the results, and gave his appraisal of what it all meant.

I remember this so vividly because it seemed like such a sensible and natural use of medical manpower, of using the paramedic and the doctor to complement and assist each other. There really was no reason why the doctor should perform many of the routine tests. Often technicians are more skilled at it. And what I really wanted the doctor for was his judgment, his assessment of the medical facts.

The most dramatic part of the visit, however, occurred after my wife had undergone her series of examinations. At the end of each day, all the different doctors, from all the different disciplines, who had something to do with her examination met with us or with Dr. Howard B.

Burchell, one of the nation's leading internists, to go over their findings.

In all my life, I have been aware that doctors rarely disagree with each other in front of a patient. No doctor ever tells another that he was wrong or that the diagnosis does not indicate what he thought. It's supposed to be medical ethics, but it's really medical etiquette.

But at the Mayo Clinic, the gloves were off. These doctors, in front of my wife and me, analyzed their findings. They openly disagreed about whether she should undergo heart surgery. The leading surgeon favored the operation. Most of the other specialists opposed it. The overall feeling was that the operation under consideration had never been done before. It was an experiment, and a very risky one. They didn't know what the results would be, and therefore this operation should be done only as a last resort. And a last-resort operation could be done at any time. That was the choice Ruth and I were presented with. We decided against the operation. As a result of this decision, Ruth did enjoy an additional seven years of normal living.

I know very few people who have had the opportunity to discuss their medical problems with so many respected doctors as we did on that occasion. Yet that is why we went to the Mayo Clinic in the first place. My wife's regular physicians, Dr. Herbert Tanenbaum of Washington, D.C., and Dr. Edward Nichols of Hartford, Connecticut, in consultation with a personal friend of mine, Dr. Edmund H. Sonnenblick, then at the National

Institutes of Health, told us to seek a diagnosis at a place where the surgeon was not king. If we went to one of the great heart centers, they said, an operation would be performed the moment the top surgeon said to operate. At the Mayo Clinic, they said, no discipline is king. Everybody is on an equal basis. Each patient is looked at comprehensively, and the surgeon gets challenged just like every other specialist. The doctors may agree with him, but he is not the boss.

Whenever I meet a doctor or a hospital administrator and describe the experiences my wife and I had at the Mayo Clinic, I ask how it could be duplicated elsewhere. Always the same answer comes back. It's one of a kind, the result of special circumstances that just don't apply elsewhere. I once accepted that answer. I don't anymore. Because it seems that every time somebody comes upon a hospital, an instituion, or a medical care system that provides superb medical care, we are told it is an exception, the result of special circumstances.

That is all wrong. First-rate medical care should not be the exception in this country. It should be the rule.

Index

Index

Index

Index

Index

Tuberculosis, 56
Tulsa, Oklahoma, 12-13

Union County Hospital, Clayton, New Mexico, 28
United States Army, 94
United States Congress, 41, 64, 65, 145, 154, 158, 159-163, 188
United States Department of Defense, 90
United States Department of Housing and Urban Development, 94
United States Navy, 94
University of Alabama Medical School, 38
University of Florida College of Medicine, 180-182
University of Illinois Medical School, 190
University of Pennsylvania Hospital, 11
University of Washington, "Medex" program, 198

Velez, Luciano, 60

W. A. Shands Hospital, Gainesville, Florida, 181
Wages, hospital employees, 79-81
Wagner, Robert F., Sr., 64, 65
Wagner-Murray-Dingell bill, 65
Warren Hospital, Phillipsburg, New Jersey, 31, 33
Washington State Department of Health, 91, 93
Weed, Lawrence L., 130
Wheeler, Raymond M., 21
William Beaumont Hospital, Royal Oak, Michigan, 15-16
Williams, K. J., 132-134
Windsor, Ontario, 49, 51

X rays, 24, 25, 83

Zuckerbraun, Lionel, 44